Get Through

MRCPCH Part 2: 125 Questions on Clinical Photographs

abc 5388

WS18.2

D1354723

WITHDRAWN

FROM LIBRARY

BRITISH MEDICAL ASSOCIATION

1006263

To our families and parents

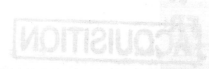

BMA LIBRARY
WITHDRAWN FROM LIBRARY
BRITISH MEDICAL ASSOCIATION

Get Through
MRCPCH Part 2:
125 Questions on
Clinical Photographs

Nagi Giumma Barakat MB BCh MRCPCH MSc Epilepsy CCST FRCPCH
Consultant Paediatrician, Hillingdon Hospital
Honorary Consultant, Neurology Department
Great Ormond Street Hospital for Children
London, UK

Roger Buchdahl MD FRCP FRCPCH
Consultant Paediatrician, Hillingdon Hospital
Honorary Consultant Paediatrician, Paediatric Respiratory Medicine Department
Brompton Hospital
London, UK

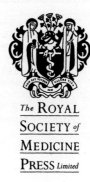
The ROYAL
SOCIETY *of*
MEDICINE
PRESS *Limited*

© 2005 Royal Society of Medicine Press Ltd

Published by the Royal Society of Medicine Press Ltd
1 Wimpole Street, London W1G 0AE, UK
Tel: +44 (0)20 7290 2921
Fax: +44 (0)20 7290 2929
Email: publishing@rsm.ac.uk
Website: www.rsmpress.co.uk

Apart from any fair dealing for the purposes of research or private study, criticism or review, as permitted under the UK Copyright, Designs and Patents Act, 1988, no part of this publication may be reproduced, stored or transmitted, in any form or by any means, without the prior permission in writing of the publishers or in the case of reprographic reproduction in accordance with the terms of licences issued by the Copyright Licensing Agency in the UK, or in accordance with the terms of licences issued by the appropriate Reproduction Rights Organization outside the UK. Enquiries concerning reproduction outside the terms stated here should be sent to the publishers at the UK address printed on this page.

The rights of Nagi G Barakat and Roger Buchdahl to be identified as authors of this work have been asserted by them in accordance with the Copyright, Designs and Patents Act, 1988.

British Library Cataloguing in Publication Data
A catalogue record for this book is available from the British Library

ISBN 1-85315-685-X

Distribution in Europe and Rest of World:

Marston Book Services Ltd
PO Box 269
Abingdon
Oxon OX14 4YN, UK
Tel: +44 (0)1235 465500
Fax: +44 (0)1235 465555
Email: direct.order@marston.co.uk

Distribution in the USA and Canada:

Royal Society of Medicine Press Ltd
c/o Jamco Distribution Inc
1401 Lakeway Drive
Lewisville, TX 75057, USA
Tel: +1 800 538 1287
Fax: +1 972 353 1303
Email: jamco@majors.com

Distribution in Australia and New Zealand:

Elsevier Australia
30–52 Smidmore Street
Marrikville NSW 2204, Australia
Tel: +61 2 9349 5811
Fax: +61 2 9349 5911
Email: service@elsevier.com.au

Typeset by S R Nova Pvt Ltd, Bangalore, India
Printed and bound by Replika Press Pvt Ltd, India

Contents

Foreword

In July 2002 the new MRCPCH Part 2 written exam was introduced. The change in the format of the questions may have felt to be very threatening to the candidates, but in reality the 'best of five' and 'extended matching' format are how clinicians practice when faced with a clinical scenario. The authors of this book are experienced paediatricians with a real desire to teach. They have diligently photographed many of the babies and children who they have managed over the years, and have used the clinical material to teach in their own department. It was therefore entirely logical to make this material available to a larger audience in the format of this book, which is packed with real clinical situations, beautifully illustrated with high quality photographs, and a selection of questions that will stretch prospective MRCPCH candidates. The answers are detailed and provide the reader with ample information whilst also stimulating interest to read more widely. The authors have avoided the pitfall of showing only rare syndromes or diagnoses, which may fascinate the reader but are of little value to the paediatrician in training. I have no doubt that trainees will find this book an invaluable resource to which they may well return for information even after they have attained MRCPCH.

Dr Michele Cruwys
Consultant Paediatrician
Hillingdon Hospital, UK

Preface

With the advent of digital clinical photography it has become much easier to record day-to-day clinical experience. This book contains a wealth of both common and not so common cases, captured from the everyday world of our busy paediatric unit. We have included a mixture of clinical cases and a variety of radiological and ultrasonographic imaging from both the general paediatric and neonatal departments. Each case is explored using the multiple choice, extended matching and single option question approach, which is the format used in the MRCPCH Part 2 examination. The clinical cases include the latest background information derived from the current editions of widely-used standard reference textbooks (see list on page xi). Trainees in paediatrics intending to sit the MRCPCH Part 2 examination will find this book particularly useful.

NB
RB

Acknowledgements

We would like to take this opportunity to thank the parents and children who allowed us to include their photos in this book to help other doctors in training. We also thank the team at the RSM Press and our colleagues who contributed pictures to our photo library for all their help and guidance. Many thanks are also due to Colleen and Amanda, our secretaries, who helped with letters to parents.

References and further reading

1. Behrman RE, Kliegman RM, Jenson HB (eds), *Nelson Textbook of Pediatrics*, 17th edition, WB Saunders, London, 2003.
2. Fenichel GM, *Clinical Pediatric Neurology: A Signs and Symptoms Approach*, 4th edition, WB Saunders, London, 2001.
3. Jones KL (ed), *Smith's Recognizable Patterns of Human Malformation*, 5th edition, WB Saunders, London, 1997.
4. McIntosh N, Helms PJ, Smyth RL (eds), *Forfar and Arneil's Textbook of Pediatrics*, 6th edition, Churchill Livingstone, London, 2003.
5. Rennie JM, Roberton NRC (ed), *Textbook of Neonatology*, 3rd edition, Churchill Livingstone, London, 1998.

Cases 1–25

Case 1

This 12-month-old child was brought to A&E by his parents with a 3-day history of a temperature and a rash around the right eye.

(a) What is the most likely diagnosis?

1. Impetigo
2. Herpes ophthalmicus
3. Eczema
4. Dermatitis artefacta
5. Trauma (accidental or non-accidental)
6. Periorbital cellulitis

(b) What test would confirm the diagnosis?

1. Skin swab
2. Viral swab
3. Herpes serology
4. HIV serology
5. FBC, blood cultures

(c) How would you manage the case?

1. Ophthalmology opinion
2. Start oral antibiotics
3. Start oral aciclovir
4. Start IV antibiotics
5. Start IV aciclovir
6. Admit the child
7. Treat the child as an outpatient
8. Topical antibiotic cream
9. Topical steroid cream

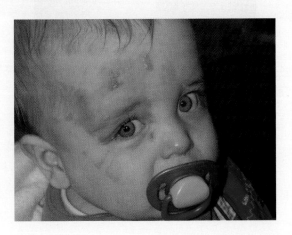

Case 2

A 3-year-old boy is investigated for a chronic cough and exercise-induced wheezing. He undergoes a barium swallow.

(a) **What does the X-ray result demonstrate?**

　　1. Gastro-oesophageal reflux
　　2. Achalasia
　　3. Oesophageal stricture
　　4. Vascular ring
　　5. Normal
　　6. Aspiration

(b) **What other test would you perform?**

　　1. Spirometry
　　2. FBC
　　3. Skin prick tests for atopy
　　4. ECG
　　5. Echocardiogram
　　6. CT chest scan

(c) **Who would you refer him to?**

　　1. Respiratory paediatrician
　　2. Gastroenterologist
　　3. Thoracic surgeon
　　4. Allergist
　　5. Cardiologist

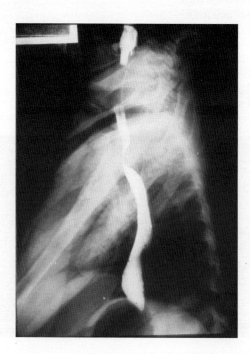

Case 3

A 7-day-old infant presents with vomiting and fever. After blood cultures and a clean catch urine sample, the infant is started on IV antibiotics. The urine grows >10^5 coliforms. A renal tract ultrasound is performed.

(a) What abnormal features does it demonstrate?

1. Posterior urethral valves
2. Vesico-ureteric reflux
3. Hydronephrosis
4. Ureterocoele
5. Dilated ureter
6. Normal

(b) How would you manage the case?

1. Continue IV antibiotics for 2 days
2. Switch to oral antibiotics and discharge home
3. Pass catheter per urethrum
4. Insert suprapubic catheter
5. Refer to urologist
6. Refer to nephrologist

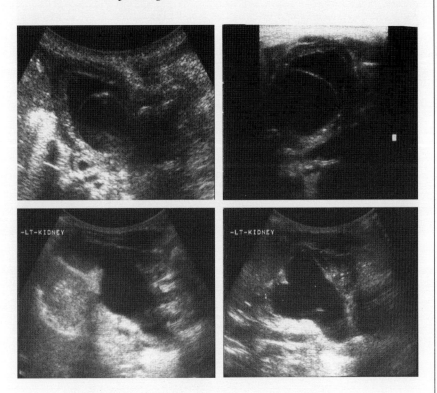

Case 4

A 2-week-old infant born at term failed to regain his birth weight. On examination he was found to be pale and floppy. A chest X-ray was found to be abnormal.

Which of the following features would be consistent with the underlying diagnosis?

1. Thrombocytopenia
2. Anaemia
3. Splenomegaly
4. Deafness
5. Multiple bony fractures

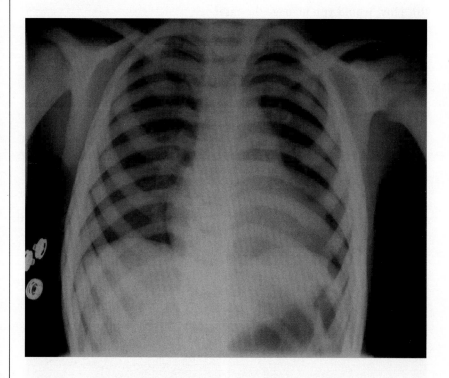

Case 5

A 4-year-old girl was brought to A&E following a generalized tonic clonic seizure lasting 15 minutes while she was at home. On examination in A&E she was found to have a number of facial abnormalities.

(a) **Which of the following do you see?**

1. Café-au-lait spots
2. Depigmented spots
3. Neurofibromas
4. Stellate irises
5. Adenoma sebaceum
6. Shagreen patch

Following assessment in A&E, apart from the facial abnormalities no other abnormality was found.

(b) **What further investigations would you perform?**

1. EEG
2. CT brain scan
3. MRI scan
4. ECG
5. Echocardiogram
6. Abdominal ultrasound scan
7. Blood lactate
8. Blood ammonia
9. Liver function tests

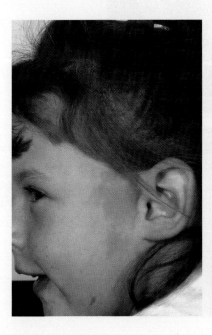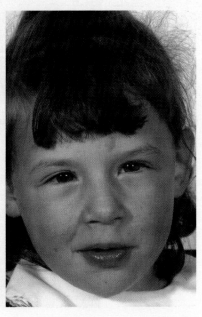

Case 6

A 3-year-old Asian boy has a 4-week history of generalized malaise and fever. One week before presentation his mother noticed a rash over his left cheek and a lump in front of his left ear. Initial examination revealed a macular papular rash over the left cheek and a non-tender lump in front of the left ear. Investigations reveal Hb 9 g%, WCC 15×10^9/l (neutrophils 72%, lymphocytes 20%, monocytes 8%, blood film 'a few atypical monocytes') and CRP 40 mg/l.

(a) **What is the most likely diagnosis?**

1. Impetigo
2. Mumps
3. Glandular fever
4. TB of the skin
5. Lymphoma

(b) **How would you best confirm the diagnosis?**

1. Skin biopsy
2. Lymph node biopsy
3. Monospot
4. Blood culture
5. Ultrasound scan

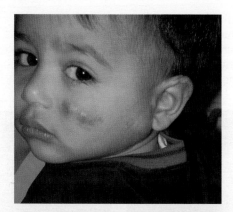

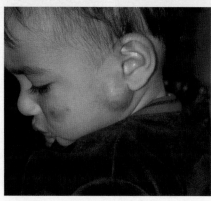

Case 7

This chest X-ray was taken on a 5-year-old refugee boy from Tanzania recently arrived in the UK with a 1-month history of cough.

(a) **What is the most likely diagnosis?**

1. Primary TB
2. *Mycoplasma* infection
3. Inhaled foreign body
4. Vascular ring
5. Asthma

He was commenced on treatment, but within 24 hours developed a skin reaction.

(b) **What drug was likely to have caused this?**

1. Azithromycin
2. Prednisolone
3. Rifampicin
4. Isoniazid
5. Amoxicillin

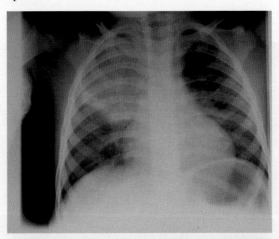

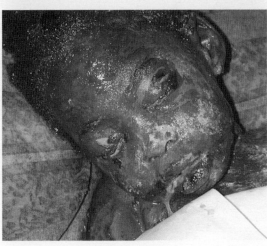

Case 8

This 6-month-old developed a progressive rash around the right eye over a period of 3 months.

(a) **What is the likely diagnosis?**

1. Port-wine stain
2. Trauma
3. Strawberry naevus
4. Herpes ophthalmicus
5. Sturge–Weber syndrome

(b) **How would you manage the abnormality?**

1. Do nothing
2. Treat with oral corticosteroids
3. Treat with topical steroids
4. Irradiation
5. Laser therapy

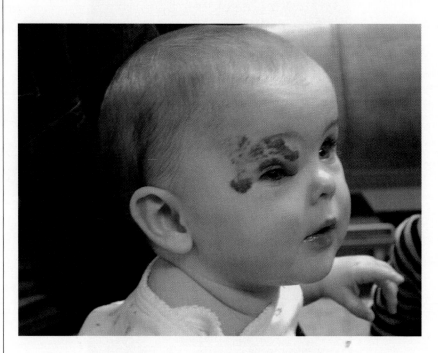

Case 9

A chest X-ray is performed on a 16-month-old girl with a history of recurrent coughs and colds from about 9 months of age.

(a) **What conditions could explain the appearance of this chest X-ray?**

  1. Left pneumothorax
  2. Hiatus hernia
  3. Right hypoplastic lung
  4. Right pulmonary hypoplasia
  5. Scimitar syndrome

(b) **What are the most appropriate investigations?**

  1. Ventilation scan
  2. Bronchoscopy
  3. Echocardiogram
  4. Barium swallow and meal
  5. CT lung scan

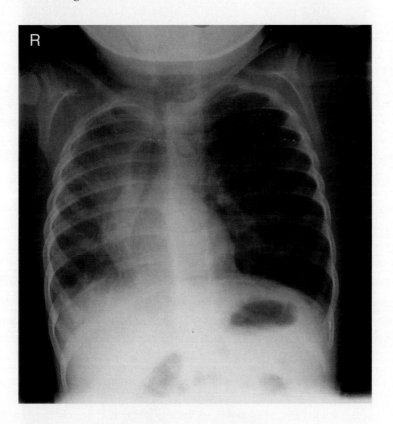

Case 10

This 2-year-old child was referred to the clinic with a 2-week history of a generalized itchy rash all over the body. These were the appearances on the hand and around the knee.

What is the likely diagnosis?

1. Eczema
2. Pompholyx
3. Scabies
4. Chickenpox
5. Allergic reaction

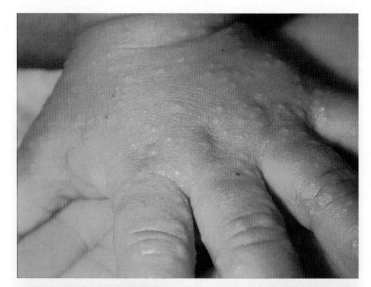

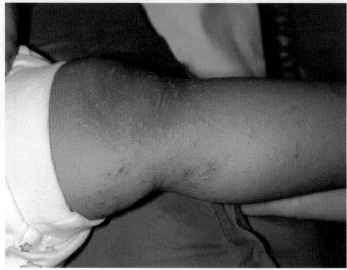

Case 11

The parents of this 3-year-old boy of Asian origin had observed progressive non-painful swelling of the wrists over the preceding 2 months.

(a) **What is the likely diagnosis?**

   1. Rickets
   2. Juvenile inflammatory arthritis
   3. Leukaemia
   4. Greenstick fractures
   5. Septic arthritis

(b) **Which of the following investigations would you perform to confirm your diagnosis?**

   1. Alkaline phosphatase
   2. Vitamin D level
   3. Parathormone level
   4. Ca and PO_4 levels
   5. Urate level

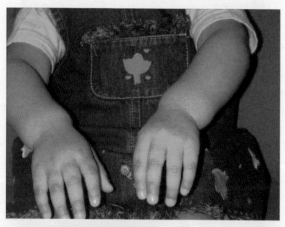

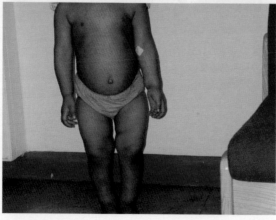

Case 12

Following a urinary tract infection, this 3-year-old child underwent a micturating cystourethrogram.

(a) **What does this show?**

1. Pelvi-ureteric junction obstruction
2. Vesico-ureteric reflux
3. Bladder diverticulum
4. Posterior urethral valves
5. Renal scarring

(b) **What further investigations would you have performed?**

1. DMSA scan
2. Renal ultrasound scan
3. MAG3 (DPTA) functional scan
4. CT scan of renal tract
5. Urine analysis

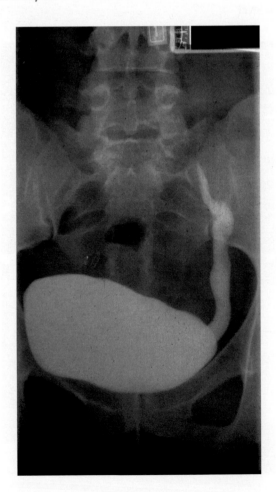

Case 13

A 1-day-old female infant presented with a distended abdomen.

What are the likely diagnoses?

1. Ambiguous genitalia
2. Anal atresia
3. Rectovaginal fistula
4. Ectopic ureter
5. Ectopia vesicae

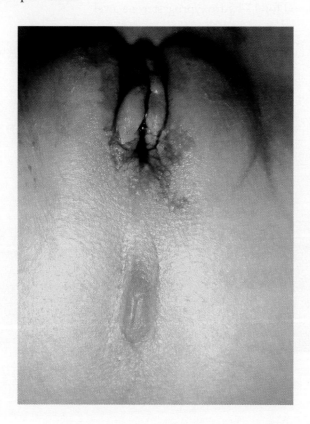

Case 14

This was the genital appearance of a 2-year-old Caucasian girl who was referred to the clinic because of parental concerns over pubic hair.

How would you investigate this child?

1. Karyotype testing
2. Ultrasound of the pelvis
3. Thyroid function tests
4. Blood for FSH, LH and oestrogen levels
5. Blood for 17-hydroxyprogesterone level

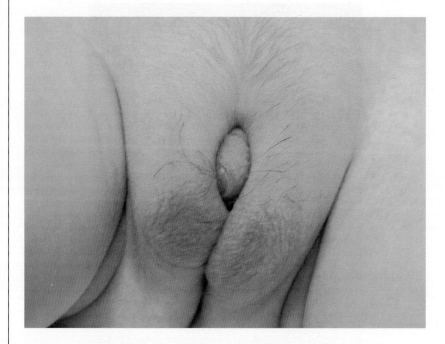

Case 15

A 1-week-old 28-week-gestation infant suddenly collapsed on the neonatal unit.

Combined chest and abdominal X-ray revealed which of the following abnormalities?

1. Right pneumothorax
2. Necrotizing enterocolitis
3. Left-sided pneumonia
4. Malrotation
5. Left diaphragmatic hernia

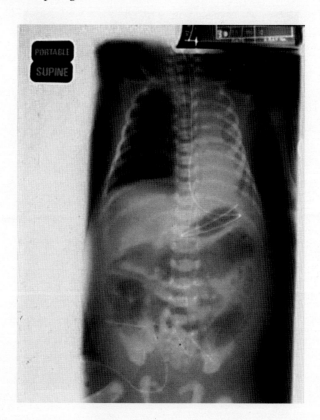

Case 16

This term infant was found to be floppy on initial examination. He refused to suck.

What is the likely diagnosis?

1. Sepsis
2. Myotonic dystrophy
3. Spinal muscular atrophy
4. Prader–Willi syndrome
5. Down's syndrome

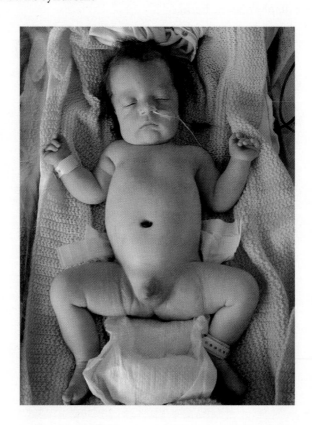

Case 17

A 4-month-old boy from Somalia was admitted with a 2-day history of increasing shortness of breath. On examination he was found to have hepatosplenomegaly. These two chest X-rays were taken 12 hours apart.

What is the likely pulmonary diagnosis?

1. Heart failure
2. TB pneumonia
3. Bronchiolitis
4. *Mycoplasma* pneumonia
5. *Pneumocystis* pneumonia

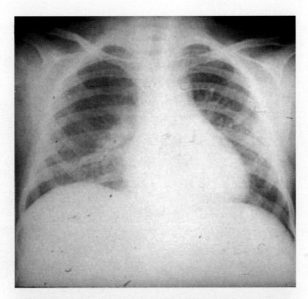

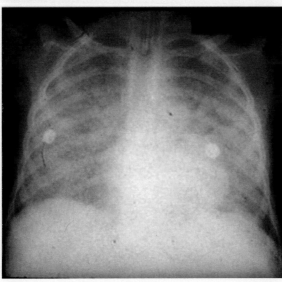

Case 18

This term newborn infant was noted to have frequent apnoeic attacks in the postnatal period.

What is the likely diagnosis?

1. Sepsis
2. Choanal atresia
3. Pierre Robin syndrome
4. Gastro-oesophageal reflux
5. Apnoea of prematurity

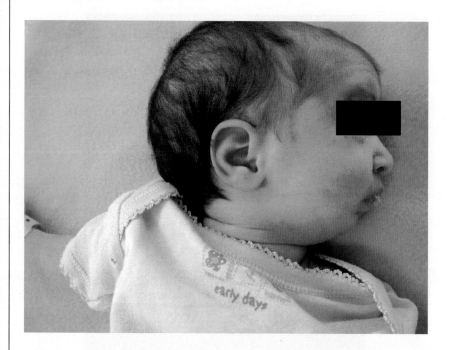

Case 19

A 5-year-old boy presented to A&E with a day's history of a painful swollen right eye.

What is the most likely diagnosis?

1. Periorbital cellulitis
2. Cavernous sinus thrombosis
3. Optic glioma
4. Conjunctivitis
5. Sinusitis

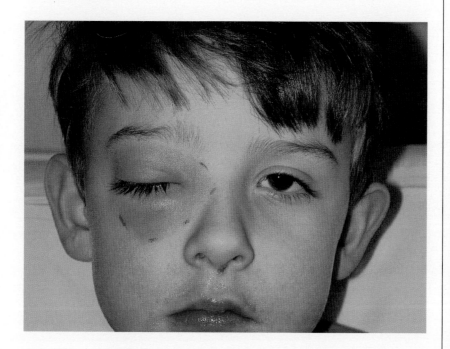

Case 20

A 7-year-old boy was referred to the clinic with a painful left hip of 1 week's duration.

What does the X-ray show?

1. Septic arthritis
2. Slipped epiphysis
3. Perthes' disease
4. Fractured head of femur
5. Normal appearance

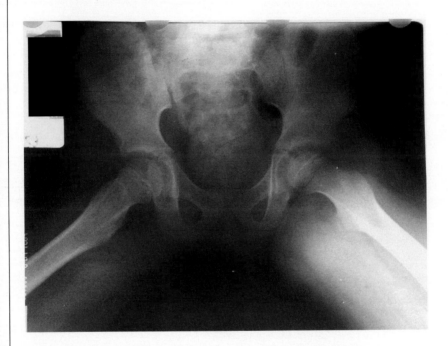

Case 21

This 10-year-old boy with a long history of chronic cough presented with a 2-month history of progressive tiredness, weight loss and jaundice.

(a) **What diagnoses would be consistent with this history and appearances?**

    1. Nephrotic syndrome
    2. Peritonitis
    3. Wilson's disease
    4. Neuroblastoma
    5. Cystic fibrosis

(b) **What investigations would you perform to confirm your diagnoses?**

    1. Copper and ceruloplasmin serum levels
    2. Sweat test
    3. Abdominal ultrasound
    4. Abdominal CT scan
    5. Serum protein

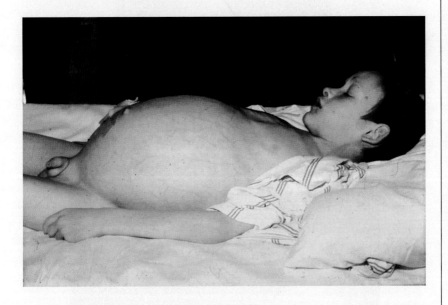

Case 22

A 3-day-old 26-week-gestation infant required ventilating for RDS. The chest X-ray was taken 2 hours before the infant suddenly desaturated and became hypotensive. Following re-intubation, an echocardiogram was performed.

What is the underlying diagnosis?

1. Pneumothorax
2. RDS
3. Heart failure
4. Pneumonia
5. Pericardial tamponade

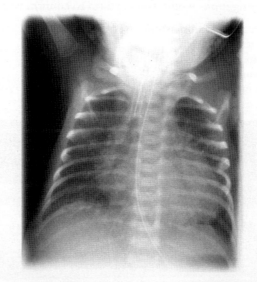

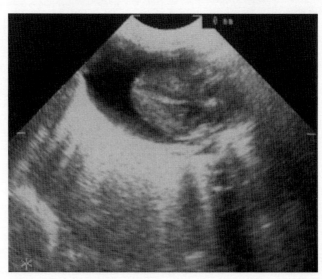

Case 23

A 5-year-old girl with a history of chronic cough and nasal discharge from birth had a chest X-ray. The laterality of the films was checked and found to be correct.

What abnormalities are seen on the chest X-ray?

1. Abdominal situs inversus
2. Situs ambiguous
3. Dextrocardia
4. Left pulmonary hypoplasia
5. Bronchial thickening

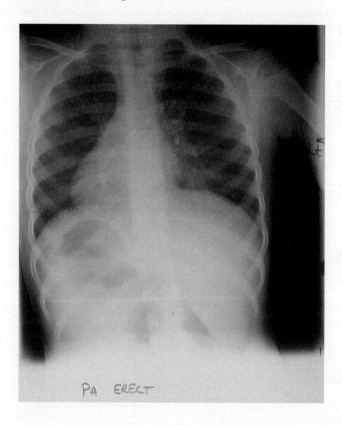

PA ERECT

Case 24

(a) A 1-day-old 36-week-gestation infant born via spontaneous vaginal delivery after a normal pregnancy to a 16-year-old Zairian refugee starts vomiting bile-stained material after her first milk feed. On examination she was found to have abdominal distension. What diagnosis is the initial abdominal X-ray most consistent with?

(b) A 5-day-old 36-week-gestation infant was born by spontaneous vaginal delivery after prolonged rupture of membranes for 3 days and was commenced on formula feeds. On the 5th day following birth the infant starts vomiting bile-stained material and develops abdominal distension. The infant undergoes a full septic screen, feeds are stopped and she is started on antibiotics. Initial results show a CRP 45 mg/l, Hb 18.2 g/dl, WCC 20×10^9/l and platelets 202×10^9/l. Her blood gas is normal. What diagnoses are the abdominal X-rays consistent with?

In each case select the most likely diagnosis.

1. Normal appearance
2. Dilated loops of bowel
3. Necrotizing enterocolitis
4. Perforation of the bowel
5. Malrotation
6. Volvulus
7. Hirschsprung's disease
8. Meconium ileus
9. Ileal atresia

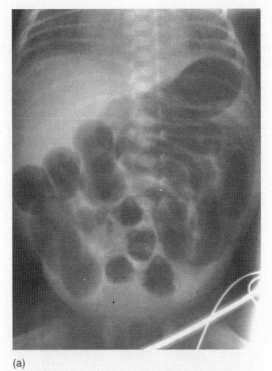

(a)

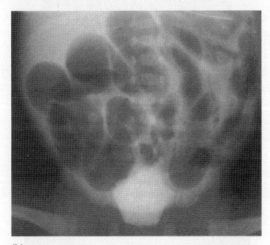

(b)

Case 25

Following a fall from his wheelchair, a 14-year-old physically handicapped boy has a skull X-ray.

Which of the following features are consistent with the underlying diagnosis?

1. Deafness
2. Visual impairment
3. Dental abnormalities
4. Scoliosis
5. Hemiplegia

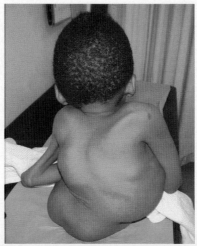

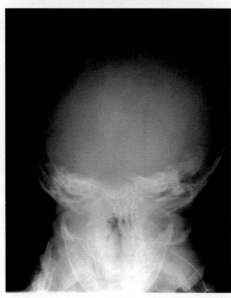

Answers: Cases 1–25

Case 1

Answers: (a) 2
       (b) 2
       (c) 1, 3

Herpes ophthalmicus

This is caused by the varicella zoster virus, which lies dormant in the trigeminal nerve ganglion following earlier chickenpox infection. Reactivation may be triggered by stress, cold or an immunocompromised situation (e.g. secondary to HIV infection). It is unusual in young children, but (as with older children and adults) may involve the cornea, causing keratitis and damage to other parts of the eye. Diagnosis is confirmed by direct fluorescence assay or PCR of vesicular fluid. Management includes ophthalmic consultation and treatment with oral aciclovir (or with intravenous aciclovir if the patient is immuncompromised or there is eye involvement).

Case 2

Answers: (a) 4
       (b) 6
       (c) 5

Vascular ring

The barium swallow demonstrates a vascular ring – most probably an anomalous origin of the subclavian artery. Examples of vascular rings include double aortic arches, a right aortic arch with a ligamentum arteriosum and (as in this case) an anomalous origin of the right subclavian artery. The right subclavian artery normally arises from the brachiocephalic trunk, but in this case its origin from the aorta is distal to the origin of the left subclavian artery. The vessel takes a retropharyngeal or oesophageal route, causing compression of the oesophagus and trachea. Symptoms include stridor, a persistent cough or wheeze. Dysphagia is more likely in older children. The diagnosis may be confirmed with a contrast CT scan of the chest with or without bronchoscopy. An echocardiogram, chest X-ray and aortogram may also be useful. There is an association with chromosome 22 deletion syndrome. Treatment is surgical. The patient should be referred in the first instance to a cardiologist because he needs further cardiac investigation – possibly an angiogram before referral to a thoracic surgeon.

Case 3

Answers: (a) 3, 4, 5

(b) 1, 5

Ureterocoele and left hydronephrosis

A ureterocoele is a saccular outpouching of the distal ureter into the bladder because of a pinhole ureteral orifice. It may be uni- or bilateral. It is sometimes associated with other renal tract anomalies, such as duplex systems. It may present in the newborn period or later with features of an obstructive uropathy and urinary infection. It may be identified during antenatal ultrasound screening. Ureterocoele is more common in girls. Diagnosis is established with ultrasound of the renal tract. More detailed imaging, including a micturating cystourethrogram and a functional radioisotope scan, may be arranged after consultation with a paediatric urologist. When presenting in the newborn, it is important to identify any infection present from a clean catch urine specimen and treat with intravenous antibiotics.

Case 4

Answer: 1, 2, 3, 4

Osteopetrosis

The chest X-ray demonstrates a dense appearance of the bones and is consistent with a diagnosis of osteopetrosis. There are two main types of osteopetrosis. The severe type, which is inherited in an autosomal recessive manner, usually presents early on in infancy or the infant may be stillborn. The infant may present with macrocephaly, anaemia and hepatosplenomegaly. Thickened bone – thought to occur because of defective osteoclast function – may encroach on cranial nerves such as the optic and auditory nerves. Infants fail to thrive and are prone to infections. Most cases die in infancy, although marrow transplant from a suitable donor has been successful. A milder form of osteopetrosis, which is inherited in an autosomal dominant manner (Albers–Schönberg disease), presents in mid-childhood or adolescence. A clinical picture of recurrent fractures, mild anaemia and dental abnormalities may be seen. Skeletal X-rays show dense bones and a 'bone within bone' appearance. Specialist metabolic and haematological involvement should be arranged. Antenatal counselling and diagnosis is possible in some cases.

Case 5

Answers: (a) 1, 2, 5
         (b) 1, 2, 3, 5, 6

Tuberous sclerosis

This child has tuberous sclerosis. This is inherited as an autosomal dominant condition with an estimated frequency of 1:6000, although half of the cases are sporadic. The disease is heterogeneous with a wide spectrum of clinical presentation ranging from severe mental retardation and frequent seizures to normal intelligence and lack of seizures. Characteristic 'tubers' may be located in the subependymal regions of the brain and may undergo calcification. Other anomalies may also be found in the heart (rhabdomyoma), kidneys (hamartoma), eyes (optic nerve mulberry tumour and/or retinal phakoma), lungs (angiomyolipoma) and bone. Skin abnormalities include hypo- or hyperpigmented areas, sebaceous adenomas over the cheeks and nose, and shagreen patches typically over the lumbar region. Subungual fibromas may be found around toenails and fingernails. Hypopigmented areas are best identified using Woods light (UV light source). CT and MRI brain scans identify cerebral anomalies. EEG may demonstrate hypsarrhythmia, particularly where presentation is in infancy in the context of infantile spasms. Echocardiogram will identify cardiac lesions.

Case 6

Answers: (a) 4
         (b) 2

Tuberculosis of the skin

This boy had a diagnosis of tuberculosis of the skin. This was confirmed with a strongly positive Heaf test (grade 4) and a lymph node biopsy, which showed typical acid-fast bacilli on staining of histological sections. Tuberculosis of the skin has an incidence of 1–2% of all forms of the disease. The causative organisms are *Mycobacterium tuberculosis*, *M. bovis* and occasionally bacillus Calmette–Guérin (BCG). The infection may be by direct access to the skin, forming a red-brown papule that slowly enlarges. Painless regional lymphadenopathy occurs 3–8 weeks afterwards. Variations of skin tuberculosis include tuberculosis verruca cutis, which has a more hyperkeratotic appearance. Lupus vulgaris is less common, and occurs secondary to previous infection by direct extension from joints or lymph nodes or via blood/lymphatic spread. Scrofuloderma results from skin involvement secondary to underlying lymph node disease with breakdown of a cold abscess. Diagnosis in all these cases is established by Heaf (Mantoux) testing and biopsy of the skin or affected node. Treatment is with conventional TB antibiotic chemotherapy, including isoniazid, rifampicin, ethambutol and pyrazinamide.

Case 7

Answers: (a) 1

(b) 4

Primary pulmonary tuberculosis and toxic epidermal necrolysis

This boy was diagnosed with primary pulmonary tuberculosis. The chest X-ray shows right-sided upper lobe pneumonia with associated hilar lymphadenopathy. The diagnosis was confirmed with a strongly positive Heaf test (grade 4) and the presence of acid-fast bacilli from an early morning gastric aspirate. He was commenced on isoniazid, rifampicin, ethambutol and pyrazinamide. Unfortunately he developed a generalized toxic epidermal necrolytic (TEN) rash within 24 hours of starting treatment. There was oral mucosal ulceration and conjunctival involvement. He had a positive Nikolsky sign (sloughing of skin with tangential pressure). Isoniazid is thought to have been the causative drug in this case. Other antibiotics associated with TEN include penicillin, sulfonamides, tetracyclines, cefalosporins and quinolones. Anticonvulsants, including phenytoin, phenobarbital, carbamazepine, lamotrigine and sodium valproate, are also known to cause TEN. This patient was managed in a similar manner as a child with burns, including the administration of intravenous fluids and morphine analgesia. Following consultation with a paediatric dermatologist, he received intravenous immunoglobulin.

Case 8

Answers: (a) 3

(b) 2, 5

Capillary cavernous haemangioma

This child has a strawberry naevus (capillary cavernous haemangioma). These vascular skin anomalies, which are most common on the head, neck and napkin area, may be present at birth (although small). They grow rapidly over the first few months of life. Half disappear by the age of 5 years and 70% by 7 years. Where the naevus obstructs the eye, makes feeding/breathing difficult, bleeds or becomes infected, or if it persists beyond the age of 10 years, referral to a paediatric dermatologist is warranted. Treatment options include laser therapy and local or systemic steroids. Surgical resection is rarely warranted.

Case 9

Answers: (a) 3, 4, 5

(b) 3, 5

Scimitar syndrome

A diagnosis of scimitar syndrome was eventually made on this girl after referral to a paediatric cardiologist. The 'scimitar'-shaped shadow seen on the chest X-ray is an anomalous right pulmonary vein draining into the inferior vena cava. Following further investigations, which included a chest CT scan (with contrast), an echocardiogram and a cardiac catheter study that included pulmonary and aortic angiograms, she was found to have a hypoplastic right lung contributing only 30% of the total ventilation and 1% of the perfusion. No anomalous vessels were found arising from the aorta. Her condition is not thought to be operable. As with other individuals, she will be prone to lifelong recurrent chest infections and may develop bronchiectasis when older. Management is supportive, with chest physiotherapy and prophylactic antibiotics.

Case 10

Answer: 3

Scabies

This child had scabies, which was diagnosed clinically by visualizing linear burrows in the papules around his knee. The appearance of scabetic skin lesions is similar to eczema, and because many of the skin lesions are secondary to sensitization, time should be spent looking for characteristic furrows, which most commonly present between the fingers and toes. In younger children the skin lesions may be pustular and vesicular and may be found anywhere on the body, including the palms and soles. Scrapings from the burrows can identify the mites and ova on microscopy. The traditional treatment of scabies with benzyl benzoate has been replace by less irritant treatment using synthetic pyrethroids such as 5% permethrin. It is essential to treat all members of the family even if unaffected and to ensure that all bed linen is washed.

Case 11

Answers: (a) 1
(b) 1, 2, 3, 4

Rickets

The commonest cause of rickets is vitamin D deficiency, which is more likely to be seen in children with dark skins – Asians and Africans – because of the reduced effect of sunlight on the skin and where there is inadequate vitamin D in the diet. Breast-fed infants are more vulnerable. The diagnosis may be confirmed by performing X-rays of the wrists, the ends of the long bones and the chest. Characteristic changes of cupping and fraying are seen at the distal bone ends. Biochemical confirmation is by measurement of an elevated alkaline phosphatase, reduced phosphate and vitamin D status (25-hydroxyvitamin D). Secondary hyperparathyroidism causes elevation of parathormone. Calcium levels are usually normal. Vitamin D deficiency may more rarely be secondary to malabsorption (cystic fibrosis or coeliac disease). Treatment is with supplementary oral vitamin D 1000–5000 units for 2–4 weeks and a diet assessment.

Case 12

Answers: (a) 2
(b) 1, 2, 5

Vesico-ureteric reflux

Following confirmation and treatment of a urinary tract infection, one or more of the following tests are usually performed: renal tract ultrasound (to screen for congenital renal abnormalities such as hydronephrosis and bladder outlet problems), DMSA scan (for kidney scarring), MCUG (for vesico-ureteric reflux and bladder urethral abnormalities) and a functional radioisotope scan such as MAG3 (for functional assessment of kidney and bladder drainage plus indirect cystography for vesico-ureteric reflux). Practice varies between units as to which tests are done and at what age, but in general children under the age of 12 months will undergo ultrasound, DMSA and MCUG investigations as routine since the young immature kidney is thought to be more vulnerable to infection and vesico-ureteric reflux is more common. The older child may undergo MCUG if the ultrasound and/or DMSA are abnormal. Functional radioisotope scanning will be performed where there is evidence of obstruction to urine flow; this may include an indirect cystogram in the older child. Where significant vesico-ureteric reflux is demonstrated and if the child is under 4 or 5 years of age, antibiotic prophylaxis is usually recommended to reduce the risk of infected urine refluxing into the kidneys.

Case 13

Answer: 2, 3

Anal atresia with rectovaginal fistula

Anorectal abnormalities occur in about 1 in 4000 births and include a spectrum of defects. They may be associated with a range of conditions, from severe rectal agenesis to anal stenosis. This case demonstrates a 'vestibular fistula' where the rectum has opened out immediately outside the hymenal orifice. Patients are frequently mislabelled as having a rectovaginal fistula. The presence of an anal dimple, midline perineal groove and normal sacrum are good prognostic signs. Associated congenital syndromes include VATER. It is important to exclude other spinal defects associated with syndromes such as VATER by performing an ultrasound scan and X-ray imaging of the spine and renal tract and an echocardiogram. The infant should be referred to a paediatric surgeon.

Case 14

Answer: 1, 2, 3, 4, 5

Precocious puberty

In girls precocious puberty is defined as onset of secondary sexual characteristics before the age of 8 years. For boys the cut-off age is 9 years. It may be categorized into gonadotrophin-dependent (central or true precocious puberty) or gonadotrophin-independent (peripheral or pseudo). In each category there are a number of causes, although many cases of central precocious puberty are idiopathic. A detailed history should include possible exposure to exogenous androgens/oestrogens. Important clinical features to consider are the extent of and staging of secondary sexual characteristics. Growth measures are essential. Measurement of sex hormones (LH, FSH, oestrogen and testosterone) and thyroid function should be undertaken. Radiological imaging should include bone age for skeletal maturity assessment. CT and MRI brain scans may be indicated where there is evidence of gonadotrophin dependency. If there is evidence of genital ambiguity and/or a masculinizing effect then karyotyping is essential, along with 17-hydroxyprogesterone measurement to exclude adrenogenital syndrome. Further imaging to investigate adrenal, ovarian, cerebral or hepatic tumours may be indicated, depending on the results of hormone screening. Consultation with a paediatric endocrinologist is essential.

Case 15

Answer: 1, 2

Pneumothorax and necrotizing enterocolitis

Sudden collapse and desaturation of the premature infant in the NICU should prompt immediate consideration of a differential diagnostic list:

Event	Signs and diagnostic test
Ventilator or O_2 delivery failure	Poor chest wall movement Absent breath sounds Immediate improvement with bag and mask or 'Tom-thumb' ventilation
Endotracheal tube dislodgement or obstruction	Poor chest wall movement Absent breath sounds Chest X-ray evidence
Pneumothorax	Absent breath sounds Positive cold light illumination Chest X-ray evidence
Overwhelming sepsis	Elevated inflammatory markers Signs of shock Leucopenia, thrombocytopenia Abnormal coagulation tests
NEC with perforation	Abdominal distension/tenderness Abdominal X-ray (supine and lateral) evidence
Seizure	Unusual tone, fits
Cardiac tamponade (secondary to long-line pericardial perforation)	Evidence of long-line presence in heart Poor cardiac output, low BP Echocardiogram – pericardial fluid Chest X-ray cardiomegaly
Cerebral event (IVH)	Cerebral ultrasound

Case 16

Answer: 4

Prader–Willi syndrome

The floppy or hypotonic infant may be differentiated according to central or neuromuscular cause:

Clinical features	Central (e.g. birth asphyxia, sepsis, metabolic)	Neuromuscular (e.g. muscular dystrophy, myotonic dystrophy, Prader–Willi syndrome)
Encephalopathy	Present	Usually absent
Dysmorphic features	Absent	Micrognathia, undescended testes
Tendon reflexes	Normal or brisk	Normal or reduced
Recoil strength	Strong	Weak
Improvement of tone	Yes	Variable
Motor abnormalities – fasiculations, ptosis	Rare	May be present
Orthopaedic problems – hips, contractures	Variable	Present

60–70% of cases of Prader–Willi syndrome are caused by deletion of a segment of chromosome 15 derived from father; about 20% of cases are due to maternal disomy, where the child receives 2 copies of chromosome 15 from the mother and none from father. The diagnosis may be confirmed by cytogenetic fluorescence in situ hybridization (FISH) testing of chromosome 15. Infants are floppy in the newborn period; they tend to have almond-shaped eyes, and males have undescended testes. Disordered hypothalamic function is thought to cause excessive appetite and obesity. They have mild to moderate learning difficulties; they also have characteristically small hands and feet.

Case 17

Answer: 5

Pneumocystis pneumonia

The finding of hepatosplenomegaly in any child living in or recently arrived from an HIV-endemic high-risk area should prompt consideration of opportunistic infection secondary to HIV infection. Confirmation of the diagnosis of *Pneumocystis carinii* pneumonia requires bronchoscopy with broncho-alveolar lavage. Other opportunistic pulmonary pathogens include CMV, *Mycobacterium tuberculosis* or *M. avium intracellulare*, and *Candida*. Treatment of *P. carinii* is with intravenous trimethoprim–sulfamethoxazole, with or without systemic corticosteroids. Underlying HIV infection is confirmed by HIV DNA PCR testing.

Case 18

Answer: 3

Pierre Robin syndrome

In the Pierre Robin syndrome (Pierre Robin sequence) there is both a midline posterior palatal cleft and hypoplasia of the mandible. The genetic cause is unknown. The tongue tends to obstruct the oropharynx, particularly when the child is lying supine. An oral airway or alternatively nasal–pharyngeal or nasal CPAP relieves the obstruction. Feeding may be assisted with the use of a temporary plate or special feeding teat. Early referral to a cleft palate team is necessary.

Case 19

Answer: 1

Periorbital cellulitis

In periorbital cellulitis vision is normal, although periorbital swelling involving the eyelids may obstruct vision. In contrast, orbital cellulitis causes chemosis, visual loss, ophthalmoplegia and painful extra-occular motion. Proptosis is a feature. In both cases causative organisms include *Haemophilus influenzae*, *Staphylococcus aureus* and *Streptococcus pneumoniae*, which may originate from sinuses or external injury. Surface swabs or blood culture identifies them. Initial treatment is usually with intravenous antibiotics, switching to oral antibiotics with improvement. Ophthalmological assessment is warranted.

Case 20

Answer: 3

Perthes' disease

Perthes' disease is thought to be an osteochondrosis caused by interruption of blood supply to the femoral head. It is commoner in boys and occurs most frequently in mid-childhood, around the age of 7 years. The condition is bilateral in 20% of cases. Clinical features include a limp on the affected side with intermittent and variable pain, which may be referred to the knee. The diagnosis is made on serial radiography, which demonstrates initial widening of the acetabular joint space caused by oedema followed by sclerosis and fragmentation. Later imaging may show further destruction and cystic changes before healing and recalcification occur. In general, children 5 years and younger and/or where less than half of the epiphysis is affected have a good prognosis and may be managed conservatively with intermittent bed rest and stretching exercises to maintain mobility. More severe cases may require abduction casts or surgical osteotomy. Orthopaedic consultation is essential.

Case 21

Answers: (a) 3, 4, 5
(b) 1, 2, 3, 4

Portal hypertension secondary to cirrhosis

A clinical history of jaundice with abdominal distension stretching over 2 months suggests a chronic liver disease with the development of portal hypertension and ascites. The boy had cystic fibrosis with long-standing biliary cirrhosis and was entering a phase of end-stage liver disease. Cirrhosis in childhood may be caused by disorders of metabolism (e.g. Wilson's disease), storage disorders (e.g. Gaucher's disease), intrahepatic diseases (e.g. Alagille's syndrome, α_1-antitrypsin deficiency), extrahepatic diseases (e.g. post-Kasai biliary atresia) or autoimmune disease. Cirrhosis may also arise following infection (e.g. hepatitis B or C) or a toxic insult (e.g. paracetamol). In the Indian subcontinent childhood cirrhosis should be considered. An intra-abdominal malignancy such as neuroblastoma with obstruction of the common bile duct could give a similar clinical picture.

The diagnosis and management of such a child requires specialist referral to a paediatric liver unit. The finding of elevated chloride in a sweat test would confirm cystic fibrosis. Ceruloplasmin levels are low in the blood in Wilson's disease, although the copper level may be normal. Measurement of urinary copper excretion and response to an oral chelation agent such as penicillamine is diagnostic in equivocal cases. Ultrasound and CT scanning will provide anatomical and pathological information on the disease process. The finding of intrahepatic or para-aortic node calcification is diagnostic of a neuroblastoma. A liver biopsy would confirm the clinical diagnosis.

Case 22

Answer: 5

Pericardial tamponade

Perforation of the heart wall by a long line is a recognized cause of pericardial tamponade. The chest X-ray in this case demonstrates the long line used to supply total parenteral nutrition curled up in the right atrium. The echocardiogram shows a fluid collection in the pericardial sac. In this setting the pericardial effusion may be drained by needle aspiration using a 22/24G needle from a subxiphisternal approach aiming for the left shoulder. The fluid aspirated should be sent for microbiological and biochemical analysis. A recent review has suggested that lines used for providing parenteral nutrition in the neonate should be placed outside the main chambers of the heart. (*Review of Four Neonatal Deaths due to Cardiac Tamponade Associated with the Presence of a Central Venous Catheter. Recommendations and Department of Health Response.* DOH, 2001).

Case 23

Answer: 1, 3, 5

Primary ciliary dyskinesia

The dextrocardia and situs inversus seen on the chest X-ray in this case leave little doubt about the underlying diagnosis of primary ciliary dyskinesia (PCD). This diagnosis should be considered in any child with a chronic respiratory problem, particularly where there is a persistent and early-onset nasal discharge. The diagnosis may be confirmed by phase contrast microscopy of ciliated cells obtained from nasal brushing, when dyskinetic slowly moving cilia are seen. The sample is then sent for electron microscopy to confirm ultrastructural abnormalities. The condition has been said to occur with a frequency of 1 in 20 000 and may run in families, but it is likely that there are a number of genes involved in determining cilial function. During fetal development, cilial dyskinesia results in random lateralization of mediastinal and enteric structures, so it is important to realize that in 50% of cases the heart and stomach will be in the normal position. As the child ages, the clinical features may develop into Kartagener's classical triad of situs inversus, bronchiectasis and chronic sinusitis. Males have azoospermia. Children with PCD require lifelong physiotherapy and frequent antibiotics to treat respiratory infective exacerbations.

Case 24

Answers: (a) 7
         (b) 3

Hirschsprung's disease; Necrotizing enterocolitis

In both of these cases the abdominal X-rays demonstrate dilated loops of bowel. In (a) a small amount of air is present in the rectum. In (b) no air is seen distally but there is evidence of pneumatosis intestinalis in the left-sided loops of bowel. The clinical features in (b) suggest inflammation and sepsis consistent with necrotizing enterocolitis. Bilious vomiting in the first 24 hours of life is more likely to have a surgical cause. Conditions to consider include malrotation, volvulus, bowel atresia or stenosis, and Hirschsprung's disease. The latter disease is caused by absence of ganglion cells in the bowel wall extending proximally and continuously from the anus for a variable distance. In the neonatal period the disease should be suspected following the above features and delayed passage of meconium beyond 48 hours of birth. Paediatric surgical referral is indicated when the diagnosis is confirmed by rectal biopsy. Necrotizing enterocolitis may arise secondary to bowel obstruction, but this usually takes longer to develop. Radiological features include dilated loops of bowel, pneumatosis intestinalis (gas bubbles in the bowel wall), the presence of gas in the portal vein and intestinal perforation. Following blood cultures, FBC, electrolyte profile and measurement of inflammatory markers (CRP), treatment is supportive, including withholding of oral feeds, intravenous fluids, parenteral nutrition and administration of antibiotics. Early paediatric surgical consultation is important, particularly where there is evidence of perforation.

Case 25

Answer: 1, 3, 4

Osteogenesis imperfecta

This boy has osteogenesis imperfecta (OI). The skull X-ray shows Wormian bones, which appear as islands of bones surrounded by irregular suture lines. OI is an autosomally inherited abnormality of type I collagen. Most cases have a triad of clinical features: fragile bones, blue sclera and early deafness. The current classification recognizes four distinct types. Some type I (mild) cases have dental abnormalities in addition to the classical triad. Type II (perinatal lethal) may present as stillbirth or in infancy as retarded growth with multiple fractures, bowing of the legs and relative macrocephaly. Type III (progressive deforming) cases may have fractures in utero. In the postnatal period fractures are common, and gradually result in deformation of the skeleton. Scoliosis is common and stature is severely compromised. The case pictured here has type III OI. Type IV (moderately severe) has a similar clinical spectrum to type III, although children usually remain ambulatory with only mild to moderate effect on stature. Types I and IV are compatible with a normal lifespan. Diagnosis can be confirmed by skin biopsy and collagen studies of the fibroblasts. Antenatal ultrasound diagnosis is possible for severe cases. Chorionic villus biopsy offers antenatal biochemical diagnosis. Bisphosphonate drug treatment can increase bone mineralization and decrease fracture frequency and pain in some cases. Specialist paediatric orthopaedic consultation should be undertaken.

Case 26

A $12^1/_2$-year-old boy has a 6-month history of intermittent right cheek swelling, gingival ulceration and intermittent diarrhoea. An initial blood test revealed a haemoglobin of 11.4 g%, a CRP of 17 mg/l and a normal ESR. He underwent a biopsy of the cheek swelling, which revealed granulomatous changes.

What further investigations would you perform to establish the diagnosis?

1. Abdominal USS
2. Barium meal and follow-through
3. GI endoscopy
4. Bone marrow
5. Liver function tests

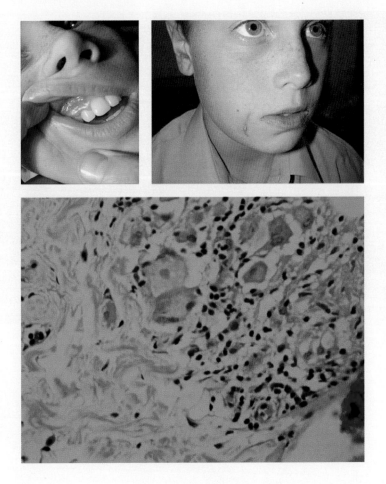

Case 27

This is the second of twin boys born prematurely at 31 weeks, both with a heart murmur.

(a) **What are the features associated with the condition?**

   1. Ventricular septal defect
   2. Pulmonary stenosis
   3. Obstructive cardiomyopathy
   4. Failure to thrive
   5. Gastro-oesophageal reflux

(b) **How would you investigate the twins?**

   1. Echocardiogram
   2. Hearing test
   3. Barium swallow
   4. Chromosome studies
   5. Coagulation studies

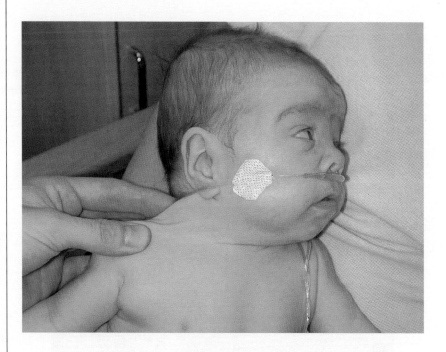

Case 28

A 6-year-old girl presented to A&E with a 1-month history of increasing abdominal pain and distension. On examination she was found to have an enlarged liver. She underwent an abdominal ultrasound examination plus chest X-ray.

(a) **The findings are consistent with which of the following?**

1. Cystic fibrosis
2. Gaucher's disease
3. Neuroblastoma
4. Liver cirrhosis with portal hypertension
5. Leukaemia

(b) **What three further investigations would you perform?**

1. CT scan abdomen/chest
2. Sweat test
3. Bone marrow
4. Liver biopsy
5. FBC and differential

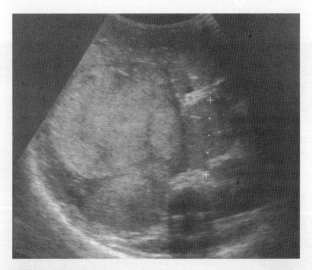

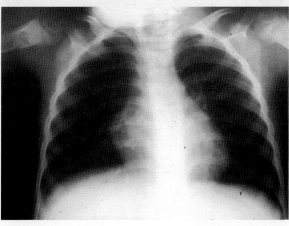

Case 29

An 11-month-old baby boy was brought to A&E with a 1-day history of cough, fever and blanching skin rash.

(a) **The skin appearance was consistent with which of the following?**

1. Measles
2. Kawasaki's disease
3. Henoch–Schönlein purpura
4. Rubella
5. Toxic shock syndrome

(b) **Which of the following investigations would be appropriate?**

1. ASO titre
2. Rubella and measles serology
3. Blood cultures
4. Clotting studies
5. Urine analysis

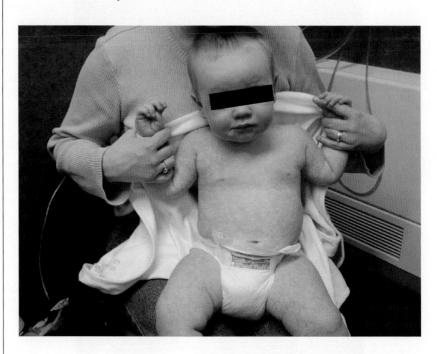

Case 30

A 3-year-old boy was referred with a chronic cough, wheeze and nasal stuffiness. Nasal examination revealed an obstructed right nostril.

(a) **With which of the following would this finding be consistent?**

   1. Allergic rhinitis
   2. Primary ciliary dyskinesia
   3. Cystic fibrosis
   4. Wagener's granulomatosis
   5. Rhabdomyosarcoma

(b) **Which of the following investigations would be appropriate?**

   1. Biopsy
   2. Sweat test
   3. FBP and differential
   4. Allergy skin prick tests
   5. Antinuclear cytoplasmic antibody

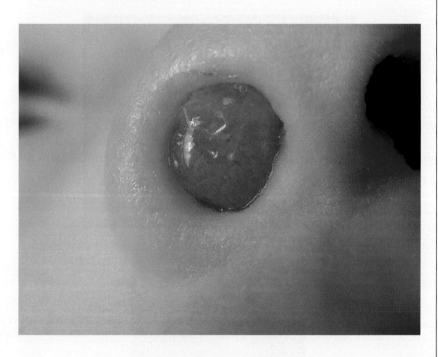

Case 31

A 3-year-old girl was seen in A&E with a history of fever and cough and shortness of breath. A chest X-ray was performed and she was discharged home. Three weeks later she re-attends A&E with continuing symptoms. A second chest X-ray is performed.

(a) The appearances are consistent with which of the following diagnoses?

1. Congestive heart failure
2. Bronchiolitis
3. Miliary TB
4. Aspiration pneumonia
5. Letterer–Siwe disease

(b) What would be the most appropriate investigations?

1. Bronchoscopy
2. Early-morning gastric aspirates
3. Echocardiogram
4. Heaf test
5. Bone marrow

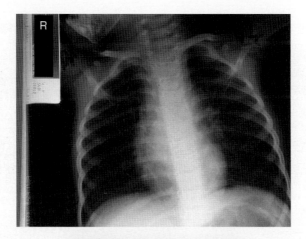

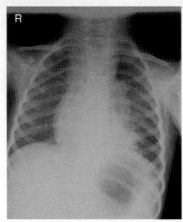

Case 32

A 12-hour-old infant born via a normal vaginal delivery after an unremarkable pregnancy and labour suddenly had a generalized tonic clonic seizure lasting for 2 minutes. Initial cerebral ultrasound scan was normal. After a number of investigations, including a CT brain scan and an MRI brain scan, a diagnosis is made.

(a) **What is the most likely diagnosis?**

1. Left-sided intraventricular haemorrhage
2. Extradural haemorrhage
3. Right middle cerebral artery infarct
4. Cerebral oedema
5. Congenital infection

(b) **What other investigations would you want to perform?**

1. Prothrombin time and activated partial thromboplastin time
2. Maternal anticardiolipin antibodies
3. Factor 5 Leiden and protein S and C levels
4. CMV serology
5. Full blood count

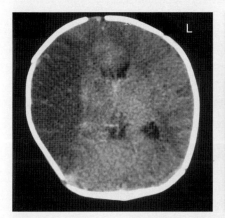
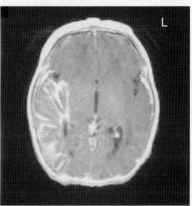

Case 33

A newborn term infant was noted to look dysmorphic at birth.

(a) **What are the dysmorphic features?**

1. Prominent nasal bridge
2. Microcephaly
3. Micrognathia
4. Featureless philtrum
5. Prominent epicanthic folds

(b) **What investigations would you perform?**

1. Congenital infection screen
2. Chromosome analysis
3. Coagulation studies
4. Cerebral ultrasound scan
5. Liver function tests

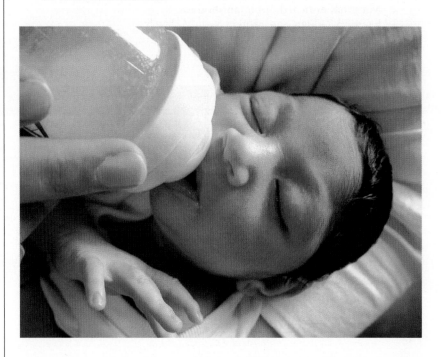

Case 34

A 5-month-old infant previously well was found in his cot by his parents to be unresponsive and to have a generalized rash.

(a) **What is the most likely diagnosis?**

   1. Meningococcal septicaemia
   2. Henoch–Schönlein purpura
   3. Idiopathic thrombocytopenic purpura
   4. Non-accidental injury
   5. Kawasaki's disease

The parents call an ambulance.

(b) **On arrival in A&E what would be the order of your priority in the management plan?**

   1. Obtain IV access and take blood samples for tests
   2. Obtain a detailed history from the parents
   3. Establish the airway
   4. Bag and mask ventilation
   5. Call the crash team

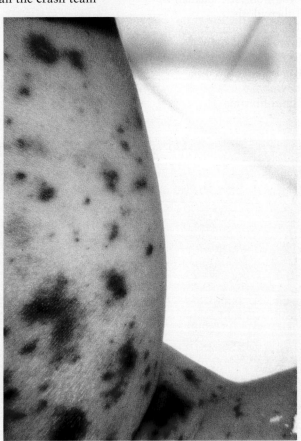

Case 35

This is an 18-month-old boy with a history of tachypnoea and shortness of breath. He had bronchiolitis at the age of 12 months. His GP prescribed bronchodilators, which did not help. There had been no travel abroad and no other problems. FBC, LFT and clotting were normal. CRP, ESR and Heaf test were also normal.

(a) **What are the abnormalities on this chest X-ray?**

    1. Hyperinflated lungs
    2. Cardiomegaly
    3. Oligaemic lung fields
    4. Increased bronchial thickening
    5. Mediastinal mass
    6. Trachea deviated to left

(b) **What is the most likely diagnosis?**

    1. Neuroblastoma
    2. Lymphoma
    3. Lymphoblastic leukaemia
    4. Tuberculosis
    5. Teratoma
    6. Bronchogenic cyst
    7. Hiatus hernia
    8. Rhabdomyosarcoma
    9. Thymoma
    10. Neurofibroma

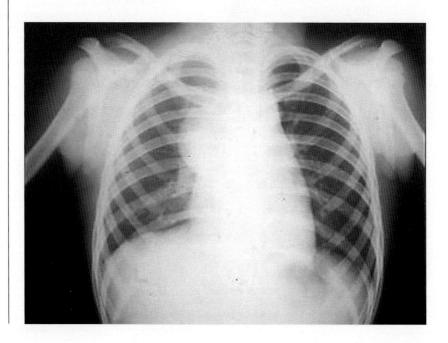

Case 36

This 2-year-old child presented with a 4-day history of runny nose, sore eyes and fever.

What diagnoses are consistent with the facial appearance?

1. Meningococcal septicaemia
2. Kawasaki's disease
3. Measles
4. Toxic shock syndrome
5. Scarlet fever

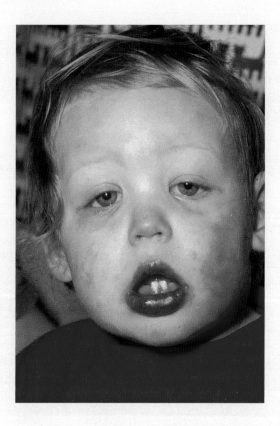

Case 37

This 3-month-old was referred to the clinic because of reduced movement in the right arm.

With what diagnosis is the appearance most consistent?

1. Traumatic shoulder dystocia at delivery
2. Traumatic breech delivery
3. Upper limb monoplegia
4. Holt–Oram syndrome
5. Arthrogryphosis multiplex congenital

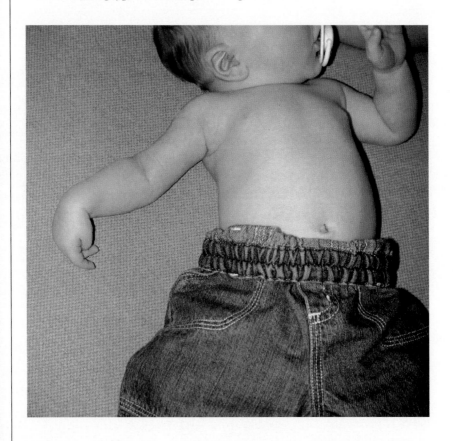

Case 38

A 5-year-old girl was referred to the dermatologist with a 9-month history of sore itchy lumps over the arms and legs and a 2-week history of cough. The dermatologist arranges a chest X-ray.

(a) **What is the likely skin condition?**

1. Scabies
2. Eczema
3. Sarcoidosis
4. Erythema nodusum
5. Dermatitis artefacta

(b) **What two diagnostic tests would confirm the diagnosis?**

1. Skin biopsy
2. Sputum microbiology
3. Kveim test
4. Heaf test
5. Microscopy of skin scalings

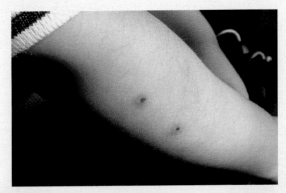

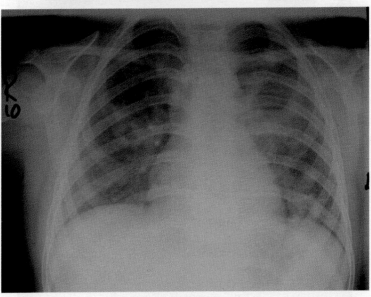

Case 39

A 13-year-old girl with Down's syndrome and a pre-existing squint was referred to the clinic with a history of dry skin and excessive weight gain over the previous year.

What are the likely diagnoses?

1. Acquired hypothyroidism
2. Eczema
3. Dermatitis
4. Zinc deficiency
5. Palmar–plantar hyperkeratosis

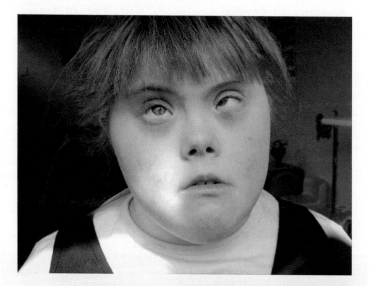

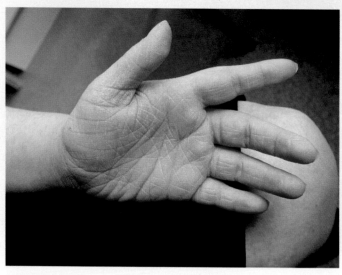

Case 40

A 22-month-old girl was found unconscious in a pool of vomit in the family garden. She did not have any previous history of illness and was a healthy young girl. She was out playing with her older sister, who said she was playing with her toys. She was awake on arrival at Casualty but was still coughing and exhibited marked recession with wheeze all over her chest. Her saturation on 2 litres of oxygen was 93%.

(a) **What are the two abnormalities on her chest X-ray?**

    1. Left-side tension pneumothorax
    2. Left-side emphysema
    3. Left-side hyperinflation
    4. Mediastinal shift to the right
    5. Right-side collapse
    6. Right-side pneumonia

(b) **What is the diagnosis?**

    1. Tension pneumothorax
    2. Lobar emphysema
    3. Foreign body in left main bronchus
    4. Right lower lobe collapse
    5. Left-side lung aplasia

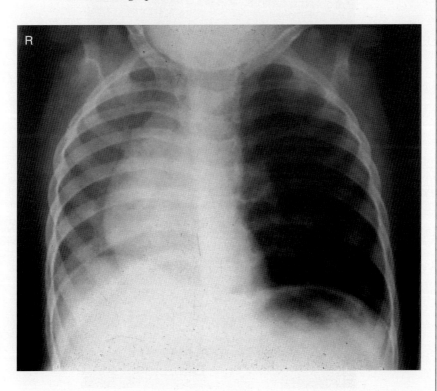

Case 41

A 4-week-old infant was brought to A&E with a short history of wheezing and cough.

(a) **What abnormality is seen on this chest X-ray (top)?**

1. None
2. Hyperinflated lungs
3. Cardiomegaly

4. Widened mediastinum
5. Fractured clavicle

One month later the parents return to A&E because they have noticed a lump in the infant's neck.

(b) **What abnormalities are seen on this chest X-ray (bottom)?**

1. Old fracture of clavicle
2. Old left-sided rib fractures
3. Inhaled foreign body

4. Left apical lymphadenopathy
5. None

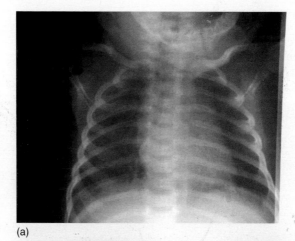

(a)

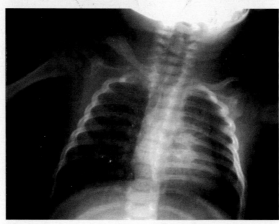

(b)

Case 42

This infant developed intermittent diarrhoea and a rash over his fingers, face and perianal area.

(a) **What is the diagnosis?**

1. Eczema herpeticum
2. Extensive candidiasis
3. Acrodermatitis herpeticum
4. Seboborroeic dermatitis
5. Xeroderma pigmentosum
6. Incontinentia pigmenti
7. Impetigo
8. Anhydrotic ectodermic dysplasia

(b) **What is the treatment?**

1. IV aciclovir for 7 days
2. Hydrocortisone cream 1%
3. Zinc supplement
4. Oral prednisolone 2 mg/kg/day for 2 weeks
5. Emulsifying cream
6. Soya milk only
7. IV immunoglobulins
8. Avoid sunlight
9. Itraconazole 5 mg/kg/day for 4 weeks
10. Skin graft

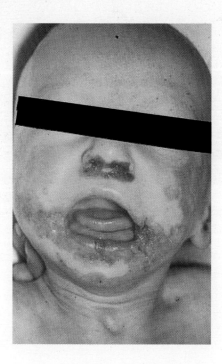

Case 43

A $2^{1}/_{2}$-year-old boy was brought by his nursery teacher to A&E because of an unexplained scar below the right nipple. No other abnormalities were found on examination.

What is the differential diagnosis?

1. Insect bite
2. Ringworm
3. Cigarette burn
4. Eczema
5. Psoriasis

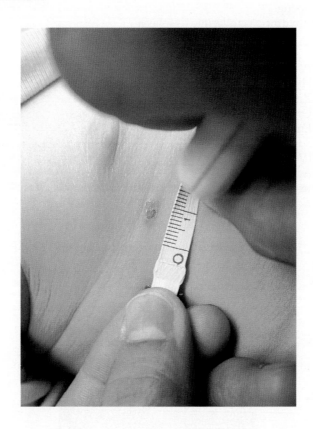

Case 44

A 13-year-old girl with a long history of cough and wheeze was referred by her GP for a second opinion. A chest X-ray was performed.

(a) What is the likely diagnosis?

1. Asthma
2. Cystic fibrosis
3. Chronic aspiration
4. Primary ciliary dyskinesia
5. Cardiac failure

(b) What three initial investigations might confirm the diagnosis?

1. Nasal ciliary brushing
2. Lung function
3. Sweat test
4. ECG
5. Barium swallow and meal

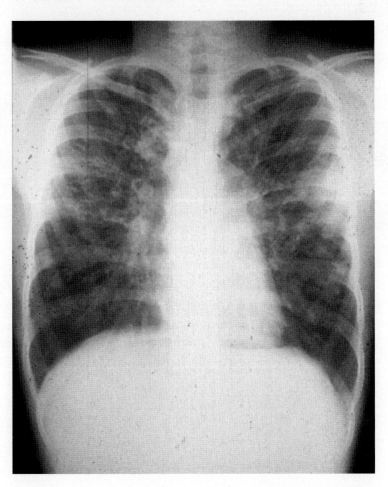

Case 45

A 3-year-old girl was referred with a 6-month history of recurrent soreness around the anus, bleeding and mucus. Between the episodes she was well.

What is the likely diagnosis?

1. Thrush
2. Crohn's disease
3. Anal abuse
4. Constipation
5. Bacterial dermatitis

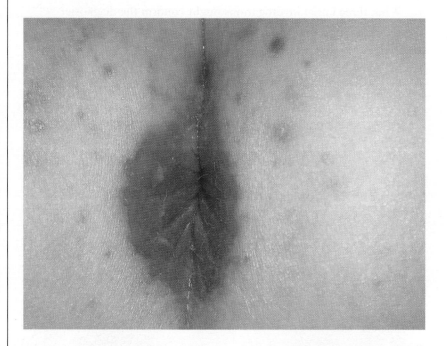

Case 46

A 1-month-old baby girl was referred to the clinic by the health visitor because of a lump in the left groin.

(a) **What are the possible diagnoses?**

1. Inguinal hernia
2. Ectopic ovary
3. Ectopic testis
4. Lymphadenitis
5. Hydrocoele of the canal of Nuck

(b) **What investigations would you perform initially to establish the diagnosis?**

1. Biopsy
2. Ultrasound
3. Karyotype
4. CT scan
5. FBC

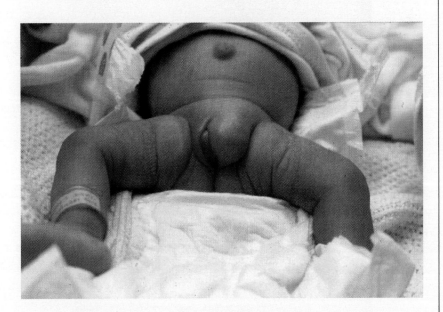

Case 47

A 1-month-old baby girl born with right-sided pre-auricular skin tags was noted to have an abnormality of the eye. The ophthalmologist diagnoses an epibulbar dermoid.

What other abnormalities may be associated with the underlying syndrome?

1. Unilateral facial hypoplasia
2. Hemivertebrae
3. Cardiac anomalies
4. Severe learning difficulties
5. Imperforate anus

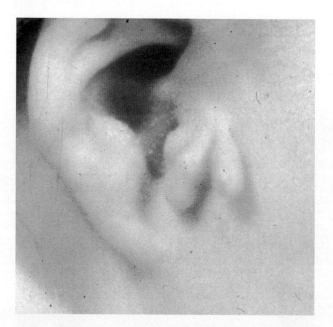

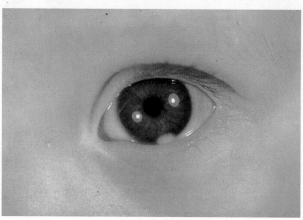

Case 48

A 1-month-old infant was referred to the clinic with a discharging umbilicus.

(a) What is the abnormality?

1. Umbilical granuloma
2. Patent urachus
3. Umbilical hernia
4. Embryonal rhabdosarcoma
5. Infected umbilicus

(b) How would you manage the abnormality in the first instance?

1. Silver nitrate cautery
2. Cryotherapy
3. Apply salt
4. Surgical resection
5. Do nothing

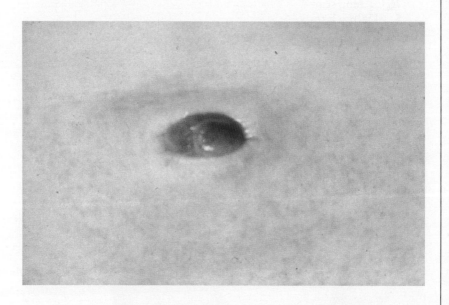

Case 49

A 5-month-old infant was referred to the clinic with a history of skin rash and persistent cough. On examination he was found to be underweight, with exfoliative rashes in his groin and over the scalp. He has a chest X-ray.

(a) **What are the most likely diagnoses?**

    1. Eczema
    2. Zinc deficiency
    3. Thrush
    4. Letterer–Siwe disease
    5. Cystic fibrosis

(b) **What investigations would you perform?**

    1. Sweat test
    2. Skin biopsy
    3. Zinc level
    4. CT lung scan
    5. Skin prick tests

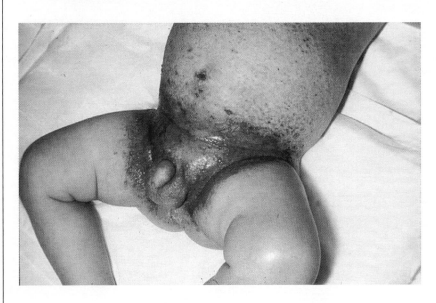

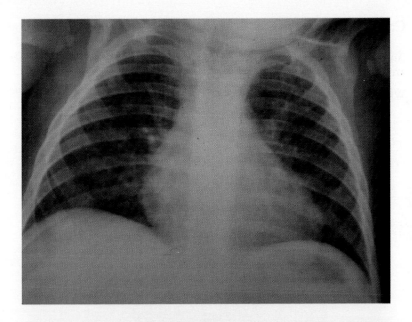

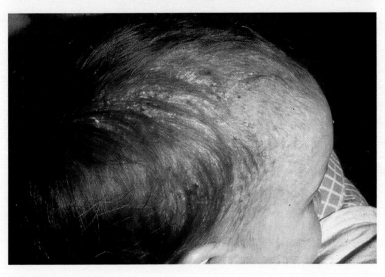

Case 50

An 8-year-old girl was referred with a history of an itchy bottom. Warts are found on examination.

What is the most likely cause?

1. Sexual abuse
2. Cross-infection from other warts
3. HIV infection
4. Immunodeficiency
5. Contaminated toilet seats

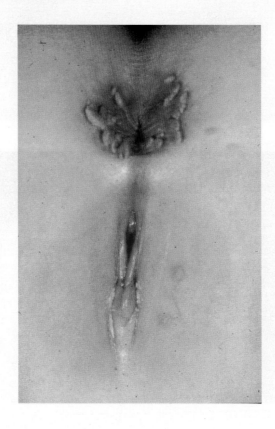

Case 26

Answer: 2, 3

Crohn's disease

This boy was initially diagnosed as having orofacial granulomatosis, but as the gastrointestinal features became more obvious he was subsequently diagnosed with Crohn's disease following a barium follow-through examination and colonoscopy. Although children often present with gastrointestinal features such as abdominal pain or altered bowel habit (diarrhoea or constipation), the range of symptoms is protean. General malaise and growth faltering may precede gastrointestinal symptoms. Recurrent oral ulceration and/or anal fissures may be the only problem. The disease may involve the joints (non-deforming arthritis), eyes (episcleritis), kidney and gallbladder (stones), and liver. Clues to the diagnosis of Crohn's disease may be found with a normochromic anaemia and thrombocytosis. Inflammatory markers such as ESR and CRP may be elevated. The diagnosis may be confirmed at colonoscopy with tissue biopsy of affected bowel, which should demonstrate non-caseous granulomatous changes on microscopy. Management and treatment are usually coordinated through a paediatric gastroenterology service, and consist of oral aminosalicylates and (in more severe cases or during relapses) systemic corticosteroids. Other immusupressants may be used, such as azathioprine. New treatments for severe cases include infliximab, an anti-TNF-α monoclonal antibody.

Case 27

Answers: (a) 1, 2, 3, 4, 5
(b) 1, 2, 4, 5

Noonan's syndrome

Both twins were diagnosed with Noonan's syndrome. The typical features include webbing of the neck, hypertelorism, prominent epicanthus, downward-slanting palpebral fissures and abnormally shaped ears with thickened helices. Cardiac anomalies include pulmonary valvular stenosis, hypertrophic cardiomyopathy and atrial septal defect. In males crypto-orchidism is common, with delayed puberty and moderately reduced final height. Defective clotting, with abnormal levels of factors XI and XII, is noted. Hepatosplenomegaly occurs. Other musculoskeletal abnormalities become more obvious as the child grows, including exaggerated carrying angles and a shield-shaped chest. A partial sensorineural hearing defect is common. The condition is inherited in an autosomal dominant manner with variable penetrance and is relatively common, with an estimated incidence of between 1 in 1000 and 1 in 1250. Fifty percent of familial and sporadic cases have a mutation in the *PTPN11* gene on chromosome 12 coding for a tyrosine phosphatase (SHP-2), thus offering the possibility of antenatal diagnosis.

Case 28

Answers: (a) 3

         (b) 1, 4, 5

Neuroblastoma

This girl was diagnosed with neuroblastoma because of the presence of a mass in the liver on ultrasound that could clearly be seen to have calcification on CT scan. Her chest X-ray showed a lytic bone deposit in the head of the right humerus. Neuroblastoma in childhood occurs with a frequency of approximately 1 in 10 000. The most common presentation is with an abdominal mass, but, with 70% of cases having already metastasized at presentation, initial symptoms may include anaemia (marrow involvement) or bone pain (bone deposits). Presentation in infancy also occurs, although the disease usually has a different natural history and a better prognosis than later in childhood. Diagnosis is confirmed by tissue biopsy of the tumour. Deletions of the short arm of chromosome 1 are seen in up to 80% of cases. Radiological imaging should be comprehensive in order to stage the extent of the disease (stages I to IV). Abdominal ultrasound, CT and MRI scanning are used along with conventional X-ray imaging. Up to 90% of children are found to have elevated urinary catecholamines, which can be measured over 24 hours or as a 'spot' urine sample in relation to the creatinine concentration. Where the tumour is confined and lacking metastases, surgical resection alone may be indicated. Usually, however, a combination of surgical debulking and chemotherapy is indicated. Combination chemotherapy consisting of pulses of vincristine, carboplatin, etoposide, cyclophosphamide and cisplatin (OPEC) is often prescribed. For the poorest-prognosis group marrow transplantation is an option. Prognosis in this group is only 10–15% survival at 5 years.

Case 29

Answers: (a) 1, 2, 4, 5

         (b) 1, 2, 3

Morbilliform rash

The differential diagnosis of a non-blanching morbilliform rash includes the following: measles, rubella, streptococcal infection, Kawasaki's disease, toxic shock syndrome, roseola (HHV6 and 7), drug reaction and non-specific viral infection. In most instances, as was the case with this child, where there is no evidence of shock or toxicity, reassurance is all that is required. Investigations are warranted if the child is unwell with a high persistent fever, signs of shock or severe mucosal involvement. These would include FBC, CRP, blood cultures, ASO titre, viral serology (to include measles, rubella, and HHV6 and 7), antistaphylococcal lysins, clotting studies, biochemistry, liver function and blood gases.

Case 30

Answers: (a) 1, 3
　　　　 (b) 2, 4

Nasal polyp

Nasal polyps are found in association with cystic fibrosis or allergic rhinitis. They rarely respond to nasal decongestants. Topic nasal steroids may be helpful, although large polyps can only be removed by surgery. Recurrence following surgery in cystic fibrosis is high.

Case 31

Answers: (a) 3
　　　　 (b) 4, 5

Miliary pulmonary tuberculosis

This child had a diagnosis of miliary pulmonary TB, which was confirmed with a strongly positive grade 4 Heaf test. Gastric aspirates failed to identify acid-fast bacilli and cultures were negative. Nevertheless, the appearance of miliary shadowing and left hilar lymphadenopathy on the second chest X-ray prompted a high index of suspicion. The rate of positive microbiology from pulmonary secretions or gastric aspirates in miliary TB is low. Liver biopsy or bone marrow are said to be more successful, but these were not done in this case. She received 6 months of standard TB chemotherapy comprising rifampicin and isoniazid, with ethambutol and pyrazinamide for the first 2 months.

Case 32

Answers: (a) 3
　　　　 (b) 1, 2, 3, 4, 5

Right middle cerebral infarct

The CT brain scan demonstrates an area of low attenuation in the right hemisphere. Further MRI scanning confirms this to be an infarct conforming to the area of brain supplied by the right middle cerebral artery. Initial ultrasound scanning of the brain may show some brightness implying oedema, but is often normal. CT and MRI scanning are more diagnostic. Infants with this type of cerebral damage will often develop a contralateral hemiplegia, but neurodevelopment otherwise is difficult to predict and is often relatively normal.

Following this kind of neonatal vascular event, thrombophilia investigations are often performed. Prothrombotic studies include measurement of prothrombin, activated partial thromboplastin, thrombin and reptilase times, lipoprotein A and fibrinogen levels, activities of antithrombin III, protein S and C, plasminogen, factor V Leiden and prothrombin mutations, and antiphospholipid antibodies (lupus anticoagulant, anticardiolipin and anti-β_2-glycoprotein I). In the context of preventing further events and antenatal counselling, positive results should be discussed with a specialist haematologist.

Case 33

Answers: (a) 1, 2
          (b) 1, 2, 4

Microcephaly

This infant was found to be microcephalic at birth. Despite investigations, no identifiable cause was found. The approach to investigating microcephaly is to categorize the disorder into primary genetic and secondary. When considering primary genetic causes, always look for other dysmorphic features. The condition is associated with Down's, Edwards', cri-du-chat, Cornelia de Lange and Rubinstein–Taybi syndromes. A normal cytogenetic profile will exclude the trisomies. Autosomal dominant and recessive and X-linked primary microcephaly remain. Of the secondary causes, radiation in early pregnancy, drug teratogenicity (including alcohol and anticonvulsants) and congenital infection should be considered. Microcephaly developing in the first year of life should also prompt consideration of postnatal meningitis or encephalitis, hypoxic ischaemic encephalopathy at birth, and inborn errors of metabolism.

Case 34

Answers: (a) 1
          (b) 3, 4, 5, 1, 2

Meningococcal septicaemia

On arrival in the A&E department the boy was shocked and moribund with a Glasgow coma scale of 2. The characteristic extensive ecchymotic non-blanching rash was strongly suggestive of meningococcal septicaemia, which was confirmed from blood cultures. A non-blanching rash may also be found in Henoch–Schönlein purpura, idiopathic thrombocytopenic purpura and viral infection, in association with streptococcal sore throat, and as a drug reaction or accidental or non-accidental injury. The presence of a few non-blanching spots over the face, neck or upper chest may be seen as a secondary phenomenon due to excessive coughing or vomiting or as a skin reaction to drugs.

    The immediate management of this child should follow established emergency life support procedures. He required multidisciplinary support with early anaesthetic team intervention. Immediate help included establishment of a secure airway, adequate ventilation, circulatory support, IV access (at least two lines) and arterial access. Shock was treated with bolus doses of saline and broad-spectrum antibiotic administered intravenously after blood cultures had been obtained. The Children's Acute Transport Team (CAT) was called to collect the child for transport to a central PICU.

Case 35

Answers: (a) 5, 6
  (b) 5

Mediastinal teratomas

These are tumours arising from all three germinal layers with a lack of organization. They may be solid or cystic. They always arise in the anterior superior mediastinum and extend from C6 to L4. Sometimes they are found accidentally on chest X-ray or present with airway obstruction. They appear as well-defined masses with calcification on chest X-ray. Chest CT or chest MRI is essential to localize the tumour and look for interspinal extension. The differential diagnosis includes thymoma, cyst, lymphoma and neurogenic cyst. The α-fetoprotein level can be high. Complete surgical excision is possible.

Case 36

Answer: 2, 3, 4, 5

Kawasaki's disease

This child has Kawasaki's disease. A similar blanching rash may be seen in measles, rubella, streptococcal scarlet fever and toxic shock syndrome, but in Kawasaki's disease it is the presence of a high fever persisting more than 5 days plus at least four of the five following features that establishes the diagnosis:

1. Erythematous maculopapular polymorphous non-vesicular rash
2. Non-purulent conjunctivitis
3. Oropharyngeal inflammation with lip fissuring/strawberry tongue
4. Changes of the extremities, including plantar–palmar erythema, swelling and desquamation in the 2nd or 3rd week starting around the fingers and toes.
5. Lymphadenopathy >1.5 cm

Blood tests may be performed, but these are usually to exclude other diagnoses. FBC may show an initial neutrophilia. In the 2nd and 3rd weeks there is often a thrombocytosis. There is no definitive test for the disease. Prompt recognition is essential so that treatment can be started, which will prevent the development of coronary aneurysms. Treatment is with aspirin and high-dose intravenous human immunoglobulin. Aspirin should be continued for 6 weeks. All cases should be referred to a cardiologist for follow-up.

Case 37

Answer: 1

Erb's palsy

This child has a right-sided Erb's palsy as a result of birth trauma to the upper roots and branches of the brachial plexus. The injury is most often seen after a difficult shoulder delivery or where there is hyperextension of the head as in a breech delivery. Movement of the arm on the affected side is impoverished in particular in abduction, flexion and supination and there may be a characteristic 'waiter's tip' posture of the hand. The less common Klumpke's palsy occurs after excessive traction or hyperabduction of the arm as in a delivery with presenting arm. Damage is to the lower brachial plexus roots. Modern management should include X-rays of the chest and shoulder on the affected side (to check for clavicular, humeral and rib fractures). Although the majority of these injuries have a favourable outcome, referral to a specialist orthopaedic or neurological service for assessment of the degree of nerve damage is essential. Persistent weakness may indicate nerve root avulsion. Peripheral nerve grafting and reconstruction as well as tendon/muscle release may be possible.

Case 38

Answers: (a) 4

(b) 2, 4

Erythema nodosum associated with pulmonary tuberculosis

The dermatologist diagnosed erythema nodosum and arranged a chest X-ray, which revealed cavitating lesions in the right and left lungs. A Heaf test was not performed because the child was able to expectorate and a Ziehl–Nielsen staining of the initial sample revealed the presence of acid-fast bacilli. Growth was subsequently positive for *Mycobacterium tuberculosis*, which was fully sensitive.

Erythema nodusum appears as flat to slightly raised lumps erythematous to purple in colour and is found classically over the shins but may appear anywhere on the body. The lumps are often painful, but typically do not ulcerate. The child in this case found the lesions pruritic and scratched them open. The rash disappeared within 2 weeks of starting TB chemotherapy. Erythema nodusum may be found associated with a variety of infections, including fungal infections, hepatitis B, leptospirosis and glandular fever. It is also associated with rheumatic fever, chronic inflammatory bowel disease and a variety of medications, including sulfonamides, salicylates and the contraceptive pill.

Case 39

Answer: 1, 5

Acquired-hypothyroidism and palmar–plantar hyperkeratosis

This child with Down's syndrome was found to be severely hypothyroid. While children with Down's syndrome may have dry skin, including palmar–plantar hyperkeratosis, this child's skin condition improved with thyroxine replacement. There is controversy about the role of zinc in the aetiology of thyroid disease – this child was found to have a marginally low zinc level, but the skin rash caused by zinc deficiency known as acrodermatitis enterohepatica has a different appearance altogether, namely red scaly patches, and tends to affect undernourished infants.

Case 40

Answers: (a) 3, 4
　　　　　(b) 3

Foreign-body inhalation

This occurs in children under the age of 4 years. Peanuts and groundnuts are among the most commonly inhaled materials. Grass seeds are common in some parts of the world. The most common site of impaction is the segmental bronchus, particularly the right main bronchus, and this rarely causes immediate asphyxia. The chest X-ray will show hyperinflation of the affected segment, and if the history is not clear then radiological screening looking for a mediastinal swing away from the affected segment on expiration can be helpful. Bronchoscopy should be performed without delay and all foreign bodies should be removed. If there is delay then the child may present with pneumonia, haemoptysis, chronic cough or difficulties in breathing. Persistent radiological changes will require bronchoscopy, and surgical resection of damaged lung tissue may be required.

Case 41

Answers: (a) 5

(b) 1, 2

Non-accidental injury

When examining X-rays, always follow a structured method. For a chest X-ray start with the identification tag and date, look at the laterality, move onto the lung fields, then the heart, then the skeleton, then soft tissues, then structures below the diaphragm and finally structures above the thoracic inlet. Incidental findings are less likely to be missed. In infancy soft callus and or periosteal changes are unlikely to be seen until 7–10 days after the injury (for older children 10–14 days). Acute rib fractures are rarely seen on X-ray unless displaced. The callus may be visible for several months to a year after the fracture. Callus does not occur in skull fractures. In infancy rib fractures rarely occur from anteroposterior cardiopulmonary massage and if present will be seen in the lateral part of the ribs. Posterior rib fractures as seen in this case are more likely to have been incurred through lateral side-to-side compressive forces on the chest. This infant had sustained non-accidental injuries.

Case 42

Answers: (a) 3

(b) 3, 5

Acrodermatitis enteropathica

This is an autosomal recessive condition with a defect in zinc absorption. The clinical features appear in the first few weeks of life if the child is on bottle milk or when it is weaned off. Erythymatous and crusted, sometimes vesicular and pustular, lesions appear in areas around the nose, mouth, eyes and perianal area, and a psoriaform rash may occur on the knees and elbows. Secondary bacterial and fungal infection is common. Low serum zinc is found and treatment consists of giving oral zinc (this is a lifelong requirement).

Case 43

Answer: 1, 3, 4, 5

Insect bite

Cigarette burns are more likely to be inflicted over the outer exposed aspects of the forearm, back, face and hands, often in groups all approximately of same size conforming to the diameter of a lighted cigarette end and with the same shaped edge to the scar. However, they may be found anywhere, including the genitals. Single burns with no significant past history or previous social concerns may be difficult to diagnose.

Case 44

Answers: (a) 2

(b) 1, 2, 3

Cystic fibrosis

The chest X-ray shows diffuse interstitial changes throughout both lung fields and a rather hyperinflated appearance. There is a lack of breast development and the soft tissues appear thin. A detailed history-taking revealed that the girl had also had a long history of passing offensive faeces, and on direct questioning the mother had noted a salty taste on kissing her face. The diagnosis of cystic fibrosis was confirmed with an elevated sweat chloride following a sweat test. Other causes of chronic lung disease include primary ciliary dyskinesia, chronic aspiration syndromes, bronchopulmonary dysplasia, interstitial lung diseases of unknown aetiology (e.g. obliterative bronchiolitis and alveolar proteinosis). Other investigations that would be reasonable include ciliary function and lung function testing. The latter would demonstrate an obstructive pattern on spirometry in the case of cystic fibrosis, with a reduced FEV1/FVC ratio. Further investigations would necessitate referral to a paediatric respiratory specialist, where CT lung scanning and bronchoscopy could be arranged.

Case 45

Answer: 5

Group A β-haemolytic streptococcal perianal dermatitis

Group A β-haemolytic streptococcal perianal dermatitis may be misdiagnosed as thrush, but it is probably more widespread than appreciated. The condition can also be confused with chronic inflammatory bowel disease such as ulcer-ative colitis or Crohn's disease and with child abuse. Identification of group A streptococci from a perianal skin swab will provide a definitive diagnosis within 24 hours. Systemic antibiotics, such as amoxicillin, should be used, although there is anecdotal evidence that some cases take time to respond. Clindamycin has also been used, and is effective.

Case 46

Answers: (a) 1, 2, 3, 5

(b) 2, 3

Ectopic ovary

The presence of a mass in the labia should prompt concerns about whether this is an ectopic gonad and if so whether it is an ovary or testis – i.e. could the infant have an intersex problem. More than 50% of females with testicular fem-inization syndrome have hernias. Investigations should include an ultrasound scan of the lump and sex karyotype determination. The presence of a cyst on ultrasound examination would suggest a hydrocoele of the canal of Nuck. This can be treated by needle aspiration, but paediatric surgical referral is wise.

Case 47

Answer: 1, 2, 3, 5

Goldenhar's syndrome

While the presence of pre-auricular skin tags may affect up to 1% of all infants born, it is the presence of other features, that established a diagnosis of Goldenhar's syndrome in this baby girl. The true incidence is unknown but the syndrome is thought to be related to an abnormality of the developing mesenchyme – predominantly structures of the first and second branchial arch. The inheritance is sporadic. Infants may have cervical and thoracic vertebral anomalies, and an underdeveloped jaw and both external and middle ear abnormalities. It is the presence of the epibulbar dermoid that helps characterize the condition. This is a benign fibrous tumour found on the edge of the cornea, although children need follow-up by an ophthalmologist because corneal astigmatism and amblyopia may occur. Cardiac and renal anomalies are also found in the condition. Other conditions associated with pre-auricular skin tags or pits include Beckwith–Wiedemann syndrome, the brancho-oto-renal syndrome and some of the chromosome deletion syndromes. It is probably wise to have all children born with pre-auricular abnormalities screened by ultrasound for renal anomalies.

Case 48

Answers: (a) 1

(b) 3

Umbilical granuloma

This infant had an umbilical granuloma, which is a small unresolved remnant of the umbilical cord. The umbilical cord usually separates from the stump within 10 days of birth. The granuloma may be colonized with bacteria and discharge small amounts of pus, but infection rarely spreads. Granulomas can persist for several months, but will almost always resolve spontaneously. Silver nitrate application or ligation has been the traditional treatment. However, silver nitrate may burn surrounding skin and needs to be used with care. Because of the high rate of spontaneous resolution, it has been suggested that salt application to the granuloma may be sufficient treatment.

Case 49

Answers: (a) 4, 5, 3

(b) 1, 2, 3, 4

Letterer–Siwe disease

This child was diagnosed as having Letterer–Siwe disease following specialist referral to a paediatric haematologist and a skin biopsy. The disease is one of the childhood class 1 histiocytoses (Langerhans cell histiocytosis), which also include eosinophilic granuloma and Hand–Schüller–Christian disease. All three diseases are characterized by the presence of characteristic intracytoplasmic granules in the Langerhans cell. Letterer–Siwe disease has the poorest prognosis and tends to occur in infancy. Skin, bone, liver, spleen and lymph nodes are involved – indeed virtually any organ in the body can be affected. Infants present with failure to thrive and a characteristic seborrhoeic type of skin rash. Infiltration of the lungs may cause progressive tachypnoea and an interstitial type of picture on X-ray. Early diagnosis improves the chances of remission using cytotoxic treatments such as vinblastine or etoposide.

Case 50

Answer: 2

Perianal warts

This girl has condylomata acuminata in the perianal area caused by the human papillomavirus (HPV). While their finding should prompt the taking of an accurate history, with reference to possible sexual abuse, they are not pathognomonic of abuse nor do they indicate immunodeficiency states in the absence of other clinical features. They may be acquired through autoinfection from other sites (e.g. hands) or even through perinatal transmission. The variable and sometimes long incubation period makes timing and source of the initial infection inaccurate. While certain types of human papillovirus are more closely associated with sexual transmission (e.g. HPV6 and 11), cutaneous types may also infect the perianal region. The finding of warts within the anal canal is more suspicious of abuse. Treatment with podophyllin applications can be effective, but is best organized through specialist paediatric dermatology consultation.

Case 51

A boy with known eczema develops a temperature and worsening of his eczema.

How would you treat him?

1. Course of oral corticosteroid
2. Use stronger topical corticosteroids
3. Course of antibiotic
4. Oral aciclovir
5. Intravenous aciclovir

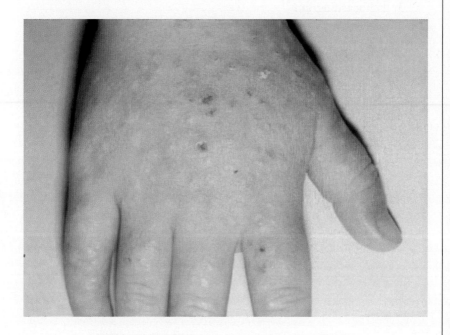

Case 52

A 20-month-old boy was referred to the clinic with a history of delayed walking. On examination he was noted to have rather stiff hips. He was also noted to have a rather unusual face and hands.

(a) **What is the most likely diagnosis?**

1. Marfan's syndrome
2. Laurence–Moon–Biedl syndrome
3. Hurler's syndrome
4. Down's syndrome
5. Williams' syndrome

(b) **How would you establish the diagnosis?**

1. Urinary glycosaminoglycans
2. FBC and film
3. Echocardiogram
4. Chromosomes
5. Liver ultrasound scan

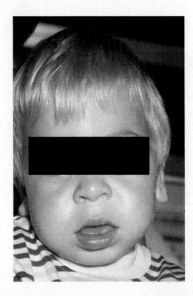

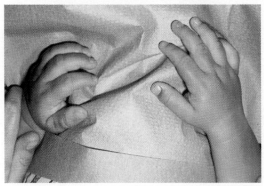

Case 53

A 1-month-old infant born at term after a normal pregnancy and delivery was brought to A&E with persistent shortness of breath since birth. On examination he was found to have an oxygen saturation of 92% in air, intercostal recession and a tachypnoea of 100/min. Auscultation revealed diminished breath sounds on the left side.

(a) **What is the most likely diagnosis from the chest X-ray?**

1. Left-sided pneumonia with pneumatocoeles
2. Congenital diaphragmatic hernia
3. Cystic lobar emphysema
4. Cardiac failure
5. Hiatus hernia

(b) **What investigation would establish the diagnosis?**

1. Chest ultrasound scan
2. Echocardiogram
3. CT lung scan
4. Barium swallow
5. Blood cultures

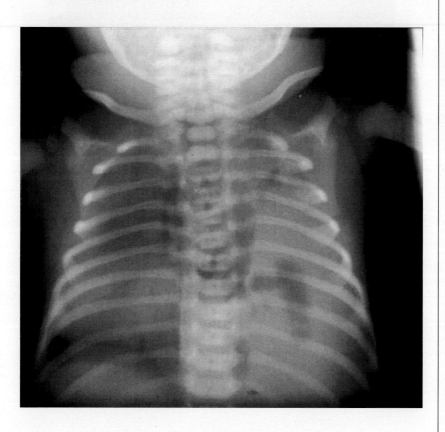

Case 54

A 6-month-old infant was brought to A&E with a 1-week history of cough and increasing breathing difficulty. On examination he was found to have a temperature of 38.5° and a tachypnoea of 90/min associated with intercostal recession. Auscultation of the chest revealed an inspiratory crackle that was loudest on the left side.

(a) **What is the most likely diagnosis from the chest X-ray?**

1. Left-sided pneumonia with pneumatocoeles
2. Congenital diaphragmatic hernia
3. Cystic lobar emphysema
4. Cardiac failure
5. Hiatus hernia

(b) **What investigations would establish the diagnosis?**

1. Chest ultrasound scan
2. Echocardiogram
3. CT lung scan
4. Barium swallow
5. Blood cultures

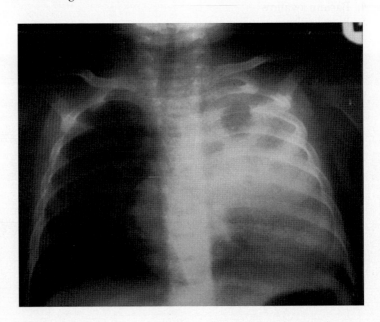

Case 55

A 4-month-old infant was referred by the GP because of concerns about a lump in the neck that appeared at about 1 week of age but had not increased in size. He was otherwise well.

(a) **What is the most likely diagnosis?**

    1. Lymphoma
    2. Tuberculous abscess
    3. Sternomastoid tumour
    4. Branchial cyst
    5. Cervical adenitis

(b) **How would you investigate?**

    1. Ultrasound scan
    2. CT scan of neck
    3. Biopsy
    4. Heaf test
    5. FBC and differential

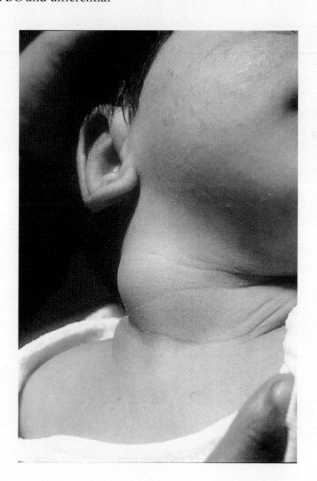

Case 56

A 14-month-old was brought to A&E with a 1-day history of vaginal bleeding. On examination the abnormality shown here was found.

What is the likely diagnosis?

1. Urethral caruncle
2. Child sex abuse
3. Urethral prolapse
4. Urethritis
5. Embryonal sarcoma

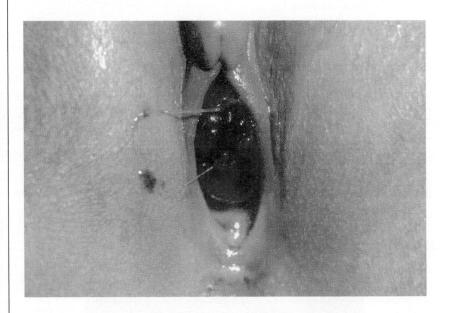

Case 57

A 3-year-old girl was referred to the clinic with a 1-year history of poor weight gain and lethargy. Clinical examination reveals that she is wasted and underweight.

What would be your initial investigations?

1. FBC and differential
2. U&E
3. Liver function tests
4. Coeliac antibodies
5. Ultrasound of abdomen

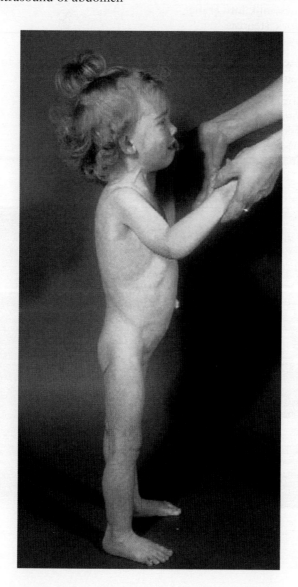

Case 58

A 9-week-old bottle-fed infant is brought to A&E by parents with a health visitor. He has a 4-week history of vomiting and weight loss. On initial examination he is found to be dehydrated and emaciated, and a mass is visible in the epigastric region. His initial blood tests reveal a normal FBC, sodium 148 mol/l, potassium 2.9 mmol/l, urea 13 mmol/l, creatinine 78 mmol/l.

(a) **What is the likely diagnosis?**

1. Neuroblastoma
2. Neglect
3. Cow's milk intolerance
4. Pyloric stenosis
5. Gastro-oesophageal reflux

(b) **What would be the two most appropriate investigations to establish the diagnosis?**

1. Barium swallow
2. Blood gas
3. Abdominal ultrasound
4. RAST to dairy milk
5. Laparotomy

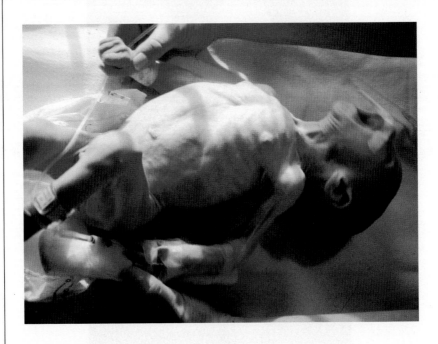

Case 59

A 10-year-old boy with a history of eczema attended the dermatology clinic complaining of a swollen right ear.

What are the possible diagnoses?

1. Eczema
2. Non-accidental injury
3. Accidental injury causing haematoma
4. Perichondritis
5. Cellulitis

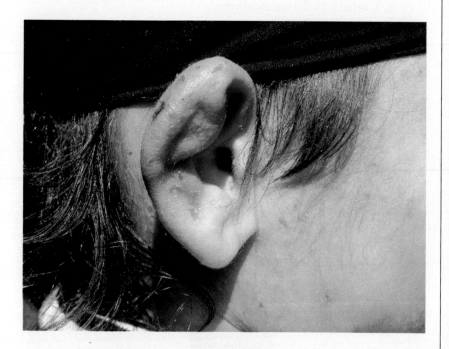

Case 60

This 3-month-old infant presented with lethargy, poor feeding and mild jaundice.

What is the diagnosis here?

1. Hypochondroplasia
2. Rickets
3. Smith–Lemli–Opitz syndrome
4. Hypothyroidism
5. Coeliac disease
6. Cornelia De Lange syndrome
7. Down's syndrome
8. Williams' syndrome
9. Hurler's syndrome
10. Cockayne's syndrome

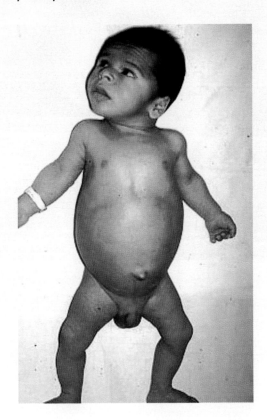

Case 61

This is the chest X-ray of a 10-year-old boy with cystic fibrosis, with recent onset of chest pain together with worsening cough.

(a) **What are the two abnormalities on this X-ray?**

1. Right pneumothorax
2. Right middle lobe collapse
3. Right middle opacity
4. Left upper and lower lobe opacities
5. Bilateral cystic changes
6. Right middle lobe cystic lesion

(b) **What is the most likely cause?**

1. Aspiration
2. Pulmonary tuberculosis
3. Aspergillosis
4. *Mycoplasma* pneumonia
5. Bronchiectasis

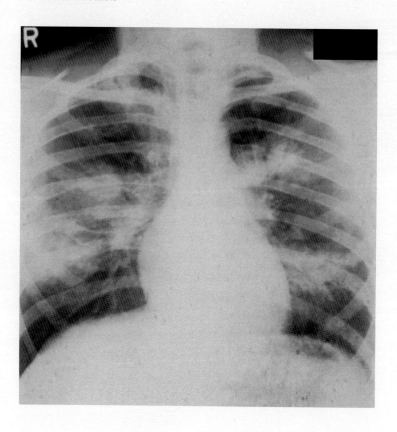

Case 62

This photograph is of a 1-day-old term baby.

(a) **What is the diagnosis?**

  1. Adrenogenital syndrome
  2. Ambiguous genitalia
  3. Undecended testes

(b) **What three blood tests would you carry out?**

  1. 17-Hydroxyprogesterone level
  2. Karyotyping
  3. Pelvic ultrasound
  4. 3-day hCG stimulation test
  5. Midnight cortisol level
  6. Testosterone level
  7. Oestradiol level

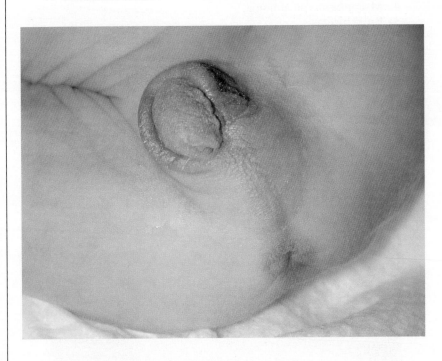

Case 63

A 36-hour-old baby boy failed to pass meconium but looks well. There are no other abnormalities on general and systemic examination.

(a) **What are the two abnormalities on this abdominal X-ray?**

1. Free peritoneal gas
2. Situs inversus
3. Dilated large-bowel loops
4. Absent air in rectum
5. Abdominal mass
6. Enlarged liver

(b) **What is the diagnosis?**

1. Hirschsprung's disease
2. Intestinal malrotation
3. Intestinal volvulus
4. Meconium plug
5. Anorectal atresia
6. Necrotizing enterocolitis
7. Duodenal atresia

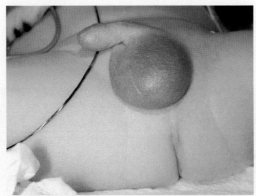

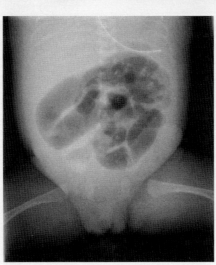

Case 64

A 6-month-old infant has a history of tachypnoea, recession and cough. Earlier on, his mother was feeding him solid food. Two hours later he was tired and crying and not interested in food. His father is a known asthmatic as is his brother.

(a) **What are the abnormalities on his chest X-ray?**

    1. Bilateral lower lobe consolidation
    2. Bilateral pleural effusion
    3. Left lower consolidation
    4. Hyperinflated lungs
    5. Cardiomegaly

(b) **What is the diagnosis?**

    1. Bilateral bronchopneumonia
    2. Aspiration pneumonia
    3. Cystic fibrosis
    4. Bronchiolitis
    5. Heart failure
    6. *Mycoplasma* pneumonia

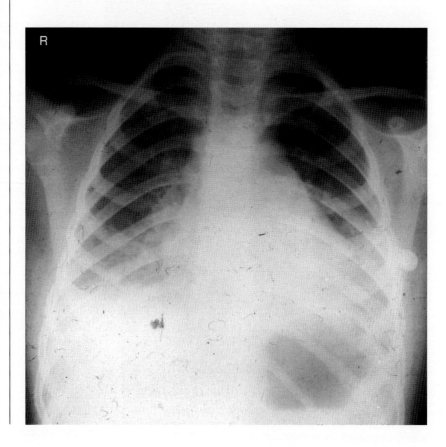

Case 65

This boy was referred to A&E with redness on the right side of his face as well as with red ears. His mother said that this had been there since he was born, but in the preceding 2 days had been getting redder and darker. He lives with his mother and older sister, and there are no other concerns about him.

(a) **What is the diagnosis?**

   1. Non-accidental injury
   2. Infantile eczema
   3. Arteriovenous malformation
   4. Cavernous haemangioma
   5. Herpes zoster infection
   6. Cellulitis
   7. Erysipelas

(b) **What further investigations could be carried out?**

   1. Full blood count
   2. Coagulation screen
   3. Skull X-ray
   4. Cranial tomography scan
   5. None

(c) **What is the plan of action?**

   1. Refer to social services
   2. Refer to dermatologist
   3. Refer to plastic surgeon
   4. Admit to hospital
   5. Do nothing

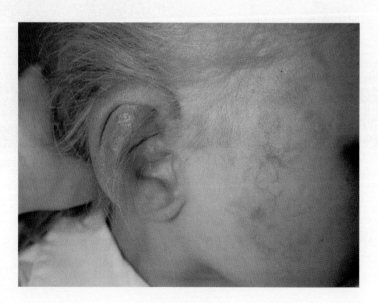

Case 66

Three days after vaccination, this 9-month-old boy developed the lesion shown here.

(a) **What is the diagnosis?**

    1. Cavernous haemangioma
    2. Cellulitis
    3. Post BCG vaccination abscess
    4. Infected strawberry naevus
    5. Infected congenital cyst

(b) **What is the treatment?**

    1. Intravenous flucloxacillin and penicillin
    2. Isoniazid for 3 months
    3. Surgical drainage
    4. Referral to plastic surgeon
    5. Do nothing

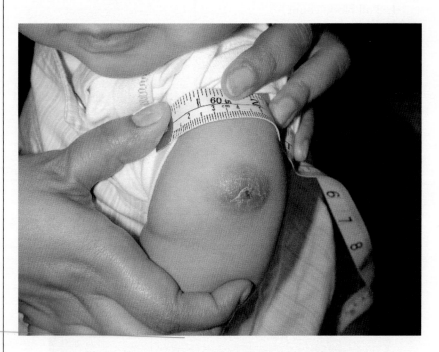

Case 67

This 2-day-old baby boy had a history of being floppy and not able to feed.

(a) **What is one bedside test you should carry out?**

1. Fundoscopy
2. Blood pressure
3. Urine dipstick
4. Glucotest
5. Red reflexes
6. Hip examination

(b) **What is the diagnosis?**

1. Hypothyroidism
2. Mucopolysaccharidosis
3. Beckwith–Wiedemann syndrome
4. Zellweger's syndrome
5. Down's syndrome
6. Williams' syndrome

(c) **What is the inheritance?**

1. Autosomal recessive
2. Autosomal dominant
3. X-linked recessive
4. X-linked dominant
5. Sporadic
6. Multifactorial

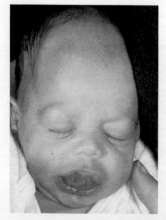

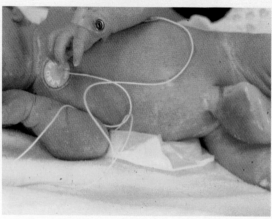

Case 68

The parents of this 9-month-old child were concerned about the appearance of the eyes.

(a) **What two abnormalities are seen on the face of this patient?**

 1. Epicanthic folds
 2. Low-set ears
 3. Smooth philtrum
 4. Left upper motor 7th nerve palsy
 5. Bilateral coloboma
 6. Frontal bossing
 7. Bilateral ptosis
 8. Left hemihyperatrophy of the face

(b) **What is the possible diagnosis?**

 1. Goldenhar's syndrome
 2. Down's syndrome
 3. DiGeorge's syndrome
 4. CHARGE syndrome
 5. Treacher–Collins syndrome
 6. VATER association

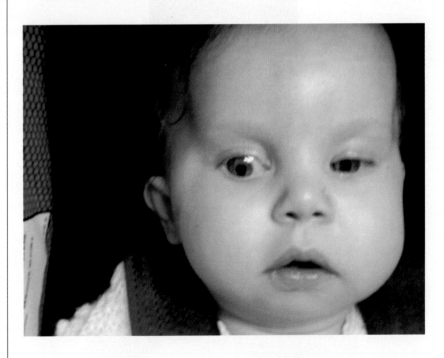

Case 69

This is a cranial ultrasound for a 26/40 gestation who is 2 days old.

(a) **What are the two abnormalities?**

   1. Bilateral subependymal bleeding
   2. Bilateral intraventricular haemorrhage
   3. Right anterior horn ischaemia
   4. Bilateral ventricular dilation
   5. Left anterior horn cyst

(b) **What is the prognosis?**

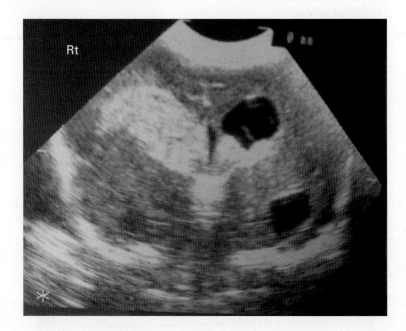

Case 70

This 18-month-old girl was diagnosed as having neurofibromatosis type 1. Her mother and older brother also suffer from the same condition. She is fit and well and undergoes regular check-ups.

(a) **What four renal abnormalities are associated with this condition?**

    1. Duplex system
    2. Renal artery stenosis
    3. High blood pressure
    4. Renal cystic lesions
    5. Phaeochromocytoma
    6. Renal aplasia

(b) **What is the inheritance and on which chromosome is the abnormal gene located?**

    1. Autosomal recessive
    2. X-linked recessive
    3. Chromosome 22
    4. Chromosome 17
    5. Chromosome 15
    6. Autosomal dominant
    7. Sporadic
    8. New mutation

(c) **What regular bedside tests should be performed on this child?**

    1. Blood pressure
    2. Glucotest
    3. Urine dipstick
    4. Fundoscopy

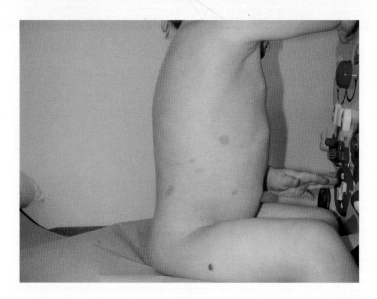

Case 71

This infant presented with a history of lethargy, tachycardia, tachypnoea and not feeding well. His weight was on the 0.4th centile and he looked miserable. Initial blood tests, including LFT, U&E, FBC, CRP, ESR, gas and Igs, were all within normal ranges. He was treated with a salbutamol inhaler as there were mild wheezes. Echocardiography showed impaired systolic function of both ventricles – more on the left, with dilation of the mitral valve ring producing mitral regurgitation.

(a) **What is the abnormality on the chest X-ray?**

1. Oligaemic lungs
2. Raised left diaphragm
3. Cardiomegaly
4. Left lower lobe consolidation
5. Pulmonary oedema

(b) **What other two tests should be performed?**

1. Ventilation–perfusion scan
2. Chest fluoroscopy
3. Chest CT scan
4. Doppler ultrasound
5. 12-lead ECG
6. Lateral chest X-ray
7. Lung function test
8. Sweat test
9. Chromosome study
10. Viral serology

(c) **What is the diagnosis?**

1. Cardiomyopathy
2. Heart failure
3. Myocarditis
4. Pericardial effusion
5. Endocarditis

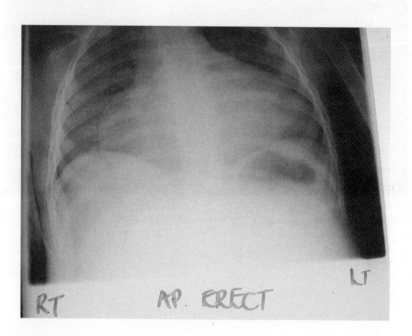

Case 72

This is a sagittal cranial ultrasound scan on a 2-day-old baby.

(a) **What abnormality does it show?**

1. Subependymal haemorrhage
2. Intraventricular haemorrhage
3. Caudothalamic cyst
4. Anterior horn brightness
5. Slit ventricles

(b) **What other investigations may be performed?**

1. Cranial tomography scan
2. Cranial MRI scan
3. Repeat ultrasound in 4 weeks
4. Do nothing

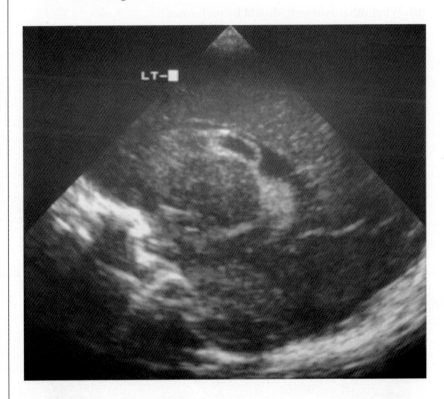

Case 73

This infant fed poorly in the neonatal period and looked dysmorphic. Blood tests showed abnormally low cholesterol.

(a) **What are the abnormal features in this child?**

1. Abormal palmar creases
2. Long flat philtrum
3. Muscle wasting
4. Convergent squint
5. Low-set ears
6. High square forehead
7. Anteverted nostrils
8. Inner epicanthal folds

(b) **What is the possible diagnosis?**

1. Down's syndrome
2. Zellweger's syndrome
3. Smith-Lemli-Opitz syndrome
4. Russell-Silver syndrome
5. Cornelia De Lange syndrome
6. Cretinism

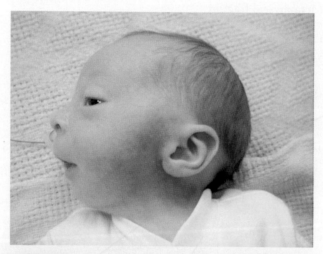

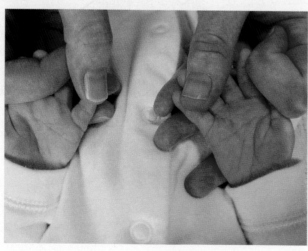

Case 74

An 11-month-old infant girl – the first of triplets born 10 weeks preterm – was brought by her family to A&E with a history of not moving the left arm.

(a) **What does the X-ray of the arm suggest?**

1. Non-accidental injury
2. Accidental injury
3. Pathological fracture
4. Rickets
5. Osteogenesis imperfecta

A skeletal survey was carried out, including chest and left leg X-rays.

(b) **What further abnormalities are seen?**

1. Normal appearances
2. Metaphyseal fracture
3. Fractured right clavicle
4. Fractured rib
5. Collapsed right upper lobe

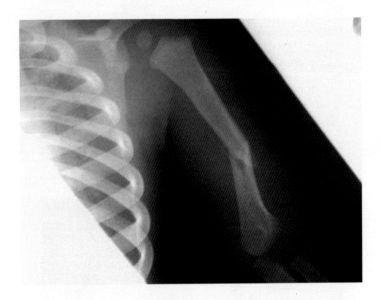

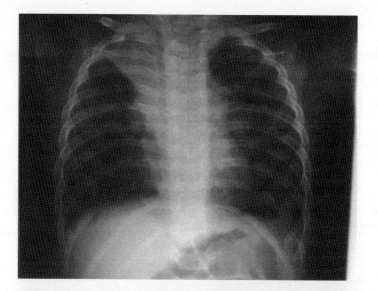

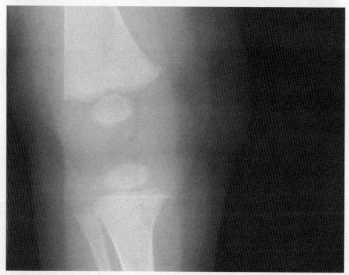

Case 75

The parents of this child were concerned about the shape of his chest.

(a) **What is the diagnosis?**

1. Poland's syndrome
2. Pectus carinatum
3. Pectus excavatum
4. Chest asymmetry
5. Klippel–Feil syndrome
6. Torticollis
7. Spinal muscular dystrophy

(b) **What further tests can be performed?**

1. Chest CT scan
2. Nerve conduction study
3. Electromyography
4. Chest X-ray
5. Neck X-ray
6. Nothing

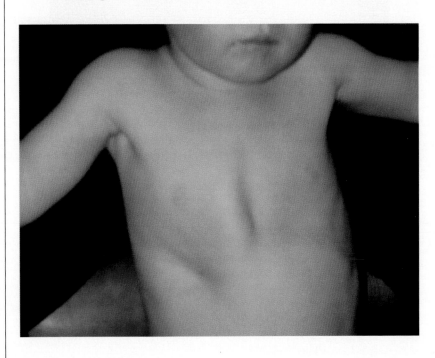

Case 51

Answer: 4

Eczema herpeticum

The boy has eczema herpeticum. Although eczema may present as a vesicular eruption on its own, it is the presence of clustering of vesicles with cropping and exacerbation of the underlying eczema that should prompt diagnosis. The severity is very variable, but in some instances the eruption may be widespread and associated with systemic features such as a high temperature. Specific antigen detection using ELISA or immunofluorescence techniques on scrapings from lesions can provide rapid diagnosis. Treatment with oral aciclovir is effective unless the condition is life-threatening or if the child is immunocompromised (e.g. is on systemic corticosteroids or cytotoxic therapy or has an immunodeficiency syndrome), when intravenous aciclovir should be started.

Case 52

Answers: (a) 3

(b) 1

Hurler's syndrome

The boy was diagnosed with Hurler's syndrome, which was confirmed by testing mucopolysaccharide (glycosaminoglycans) excretion in the urine. The finding of deficient α-iduronidase from skin fibroblasts defined the type of mucopolysaccharidosis. Following diagnosis, management is multidisciplinary, involving specialist paediatric orthopaedic, ophthalmology, cardiac and ENT departments. Affected children require speech and language support because of the chronic hearing problems. Few children survive beyond 10 years of age. Marrow transplantation has been successful in a few cases, although skeletal and eye disease progression does not seem to be affected. Specific enzyme replacement is experimental.

Case 53

Answers: (a) 2
         (b) 3

Congenital diaphragmatic hernia

The chest X-ray shows that the trachea and mediastinum along with the heart are shifted into the right hemithorax. There appear to be air-filled loops of bowel in the middle and to the left side, with absence of the left diaphragm. The most likely diagnosis is a left-sided diaphragmatic hernia, and this was confirmed by a CT scan of the chest. Eighty percent of diaphragmatic hernias are left-sided, usually through a posterolateral defect in the diaphragm. There is usually a degree of pulmonary hypoplasia not only on the affected side but also in the contralateral lung. Following diaphragmatic repair, this can complicate postnatal management in terms of gas exchange. Such infants often develop severe pulmonary hypertension and require intensive ventilatory support with nitric oxide pulmonary dilator therapy and sometimes ECMO. In addition, the intestine is inevitably malrotated and needs realignment and fixation. Not all diaphragmatic hernias are identified on antenatal screening. It is important to recognize the signs of a hernia at birth – persistent cyanosis, asymmetrical chest wall expansion and dimished breath sounds on the affected side. There may be a scaphoid abdominal recess. Bag and mask resuscitation is counterproductive because swallowed air will worsen the respiratory compromise. Early intubation and ventilation with a wide-bore nasogastric tube in position, on free drainage, should be established prior to referral to a paediatric specialist surgical unit.

Case 54

Answers: (a) 1
         (b) 3, 5

Staphylococcal pneumatocoeles

While a congenital diaphragmatic hernia may present later than in the neonatal period, this is unusual. The chest X-ray of this infant shows the left diaphragm to be present. There are air-filled spaces present in the left hemithorax, and in the absence of significant mediastinal collapse the appearances are suggestive of lung cysts. The clinical context is of a sick septic infant. Blood cultures confirmed *Staphylococcus aureus* infection. A CT scan confirmed the presence of pneumatocoeles with a small pneumothorax. Surgical emphysema can also be seen over the back. He received 2 weeks of intravenous flucloxacillin treatment and made a good recovery. Follow-up CT scanning of his chest revealed normal lungs. There was no evidence of congenital cystic malformation or lobar emphysema, which may become infected at any time during life.

Case 55

Answers: (a) 3
      (b) 1

Sternomastoid tumour

A sternomastoid tumour is probably caused by fibrosis following muscle necrosis, not as a result of direct trauma to the neck itself but after venous occlusion in the neck during delivery. This may explain why the swelling may not appear until after a week of life. There may be associated muscle contraction on the affected side causing torticollis. Simple gentle stretching and neck rotation manouvres are all that is usually required, with the help of a physiotherapist. Most tumours resolve by 6 months of age, but if the torticollis remains beyond 6 months then referral to a paediatric surgical or specialist or craniofacial unit is indicated.

Case 56

Answer: 3

Urethral prolapse

Urethral prolapse may easily be misdiagnosed as genital trauma following sexual abuse. It is important to examine the anogenital region thoroughly, and this is usually best done under general anaesthesia. Asymptomatic urethral prolapse is commoner than recognized. The prolapse may be treated with topical oestrogen cream over a 3-week period, which improves the strength of the urethral wall. For recurrent prolapse that fails to respond or where haemorrhaging is severe, surgical resection is indicated.

Case 57

Answer: 1, 2, 3, 4

Coeliac disease

This girl underwent all of the above blood tests. Her anti-transglutaminase antibody was high, suggesting coeliac disease, which was subsequently confirmed with the finding of total villous atrophy on a jejunal biopsy. The incidence of coeliac disease is thought to be higher than previously recorded, with many asymptomatic cases. Overall, between 1 in 100 and 1 in 300 cases identified through screening programmes have been found to have positive small-bowel biopsies. Lifelong treatment with a gluten-free diet will improve growth and alleviate symptoms and prevent long-term complications such as the development of autoimmune diseases, type 1 diabetes and non-Hodgkin's lymphoma.

Case 58

Answers: (a) 4

         (b) 2, 3

Pyloric stenosis

Venous blood gas analysis revealed pH 7.71, $pCO_2 = 5.1$ kPa, $pO_2 = 4.2$ kPa, BE $= +35$ mmol/l, i.e. metabolic alkalosis. The diagnosis was pyloric stenosis, which was confirmed on ultrasound of the abdomen. The parents of this infant were educationally subnormal and the community follow-up had been inadequate. The diagnosis of pyloric stenosis is usually made on the basis of a history of projectile vomiting in early infancy together with the finding on examination of a palpable thickened pylorus ('pyloric tumor'). Abdominal ultrasound is not usually required but was done in this case, as the findings were so gross. The acid loss through vomiting causes a metabolic alkalosis, low chloride level and compensatory hypokalaemia. After rehydration and restoration of normal electrolytes, the treatment is surgical, with a pyloromyectomy. The outcome is usually unremarkable.

Case 59

Answer: 1, 2, 3, 4, 5

Possible non-accidental injury

The exact cause of the ear swelling could not be ascertained. From the history, the boy himself claimed he had run into a football post while playing as goalkeeper 2 weeks previously. The school authorities could not corroborate this account. The dermatologist felt that the swelling was caused by secondary infection of eczema causing a perichondritis. The ENT surgeon felt that the swelling was caused by haematoma. Further investigations by social services concluded that the boy's overall care at home was inadequate, and he was placed on the Child Protection Register.

Case 60

Answer: 4

Congenital hypothyroidism

In early infant life babies with hypothyroidism are usually asymptomatic and show no clinical signs. Important features include umbilical hernia, wide posterior fontanelles, goitre at birth or later, placidity, sleepiness, poor feeding, constipation, hypothermia, peripheral cyanosis, oedema and prolonged physiological jaundice. More specific features include coarse facial features, dry skin, large tongue, hoarse cry and low hairline, which are all late signs. Causes of congenital hypothyroidism are thyroid dysgenesis, dyshormonogenesis and hypothalamopituitary congenital hypothyroidism. FSH and T_4 levels will be low in dysgenesis and dyshormonogenesis cases. Screening is to detect hypothyroidism, as treating these conditions early will have a benefit on the child's life. However, no screening program is 100% specific and sensitive.

Case 61

Answers: (a) 3, 4
(b) 3

Bronchopulmonary aspergillosis

Cystic fibrosis is inherited as an autosomal recessive disorder with an incidence of 1 in 2500 live Caucasian births. It affects many organs in the body containing chloride-secreting epithelia, including the lungs, pancreas, liver, gut and male genital tract. The main impact of the disease is on the airways, which, because of mucus plugging and sticky secretions, are prone to obstruction with secondary bacterial infection causing bronchiectasis, cyst formation and eventual end-stage respiratory disease. Bronchopulmonary aspergillosis is a condition seen in up to 30% of CF patients and is usually caused by the fungus *Aspergillus fumigatus*, which induces an allergic inflammatory reaction. The condition presents with cough exacerbation, wheezing, sometimes fever and chest pain. It may have the typical radiological appearance as seen on this boy's chest X-ray. Diagnosis is confirmed by measuring high levels of total IgE and specific antibodies to *Aspergillus*. Treatment is usually with systemic corticosteroids and oral antifungal medicine such as itraconazole.

Case 62

Answers: (a) 1
(b) 1, 2, 3

Adrenogenital syndrome

There are three enzymes involved in causing ambiguous genitalia. 21-Hydroxylase deficiency may cause simple virilization or salt-wasting syndrome. There is usually female karyotyping. Males appear normal at birth but present with penile enlargement, rapid growth and advanced skeletal maturation within the first few years of life. The testes are small. Salt wasting usually presents early in both sexes with ambiguous genitalia. 17-Hydroxyprogesterone levels are high in 21-hydroxylase deficiency, but should always be measured at the end of the first week as levels may be high in the first few days of life. 11β-Hydroxylase deficiency is similar to 21-hydroxylase deficiency, with hypertension, and hypokalaemic alkalosis is common. 3β-Hydroxysteroid dehydrogenase deficiency is also associated with ambiguous genitalia in both males and females at birth. Salt wasting can also be very severe. 17α-Hydroxylase deficiency is associated in males with ambiguous genitalia or inadequate virilization at puberty with gynaecomastia, while females with this deficiency usually present with failure of puberty and primary amenorrhoea.

Case 63

Answers: (a) 3, 4
      (b) 5

Anorectal atresia

This is associated with a number of syndromes, include VATER, but can be just a single anomaly. The baby usually fails to pass meconium and has a distended abdomen since birth. Following that, the baby may start vomiting if the condition is not recognized earlier. Clinical examination of babies in the first 4–6 hours should include looking at anal patency. When the condition is discovered, the baby should be kept nil per mouth, and surgical referral is important. See also case 13.

Case 64

Answers: (a) 1, 4
      (b) 2

Aspiration pneumonia

This may occur in infants or babies with swallowing problems. Children with choking episodes or cough during feeding need to be investigated for possible aspiration. Recurrent aspiration will cause damage to the lungs. Videofluoroscopy performed by a speech therapist is the way to find out. Bronchoscopy and analysis of tracheal secretions for lipid macrophages is the other way to do this. These children should be protected – either feed by nasogastric tube or consider gastrostomy feeding. Children with gastro-oesophageal reflux with possible aspiration can be treated with anti-reflux drugs, but if recurrent aspiration still occurs then Nissan's fundoplication will be the cure. This condition mainly occurs in children with severe neurological problems. Near-drowning may also cause aspiration pneumonia. It may occur in newborns with meconium aspiration syndrome or before, during or after labour.

Case 65

Answers: (a) 3
      (b) 5
      (c) 2

Arteriovenous malformation

This is usually present as enlarged visible blood vessels with pale atrophic skin. It can occur anywhere on the body. It is associated with Klippel–Trenaunay syndrome and Parker–Weber syndrome, but can occur on its own. Progressive hypertrophy, which may lead to heart failure, may accompany arteriovenous malformations.

Case 66

Answers: (a)   3

           (b)   2, 3

Post BCG vaccination

Large ulcers and abscesses are most commonly caused by faulty injection technique where all or part of the dose is injected deeply (subcutaneously instead of intradermally). Another complication of BCG vaccine is the formation of keloids related to vaccine injected into sites other than the mid-upper arm or the thigh. Lymphadenitis with or without suppuration is another complication, although it occurs very rarely.

Case 67

Answers: (a)   4

           (b)   3

           (c)   5

Beckwith–Wiedemann syndrome

This is mostly sporadic but can be autosomal recessive. The features of this syndrome include macrosomia and macroglossia with difficulty in feeding. There are linear fissures in the lobules of the external ears, renal dysplasia with enlarged or abnormal kidneys, and pancreatic hyperplasia, which is the cause of the hypoglycaemia associated with this syndrome. Interstitial cell hyperplasia of gonads, pituitary hyperplasia, diaphragmatic eventration, cryptorchidism and fetal adrenocortical cytomegaly are other features associated with Beckwith–Wiedemann syndrome. Omphalocoele or umbilical abnormalities can be noticed at birth or antenatally. Prediabetic older patients, occasional hepatomegaly, thyroid or thymic enlargement, skeletal asymmetry, micro- or hydrocephaly, and uterine abnormalities may occur with this syndrome. The gene is located on chromosome 11, which is also associated with Wilms' tumour and aniridia. Mental retardation is usually mild to moderate, and treating hypoglycaemia has a great impact on future cognitive development.

Case 68

Answers: (a)   3, 5

           (b)   4

CHARGE syndrome

This is usually associated with **c**oloboma of the iris, which is usually inferomedial, **h**eart defects, **a**tresia of the choanae, **r**etarded growth development, **g**enital abnormalities, and **e**ar or hearing problems.

Case 69

Answers: (a) 2, 4

(b) Risk of left-sided hemiplegia and post-haemorrhagic hydro-cephalus

Intraventricular haemorrhage

The prognosis following IVH can be explained to parents according to the type of bleeding and other associated factors. Premature babies are at risk of developing intraventricular haemorrhages. There are different types of classi-fication of IVH. In general, it is best to describe the position and extent of the haemorrhage. Minor haemorrhages include subependymal haemorrhages. A major haemorrhage will include bleeding into the ventricular space with dilatation. The most severe haemorrhages are those, into the substance of the brain itself ('parenchymatous'); these can progress to cystic leucomalacia. There are risk factors that contribute to IVH in preterm babies, namely gesta-tional age, birth weight, respiratory distress syndrome, artificial ventilation, hypercarbia, pneumothorax and necrotizing enterocolitis. The presence of any of these increases the risk of IVH in preterm babies.

Case 70

Answers: (a) 2, 3, 4, 5

(b) 4, 6

(c) 1, 4

Complications of neurofibromatosis

Diagnosing neurofibromatosis type I (NFI) is based on history and clinical examination. The presence of café-au-lait spots is a must (six of >6 mm in prepubertal and >15 mm in pubertal patients). Then three out of the following: axillary flickering, familial history, optic glioma, plexiform neurofibroma, bone abnormalities (pseudoarthrosis, hydrocephalus, kyphosis) and renal problems (polycystic, renal artery stenosis, high blood pressure).

Other complications of NFI are epilepsy, bony lesions, mental retardation, dementia, paraplegia, tumours, meningioma, neuroblastoma, phaeochromocy-toma, glaucoma, megacolon, phakoma, and neural crest tumour with raised vanillylmandelic acid. The defective gene is located on chromosome 17 (while that for NF2 is located on chromosome 22).

Case 71

Answers: (a) 3
       (b) 4, 5
       (c) 1

Dilated cardiomyopathy

This is characterized by impaired systolic function of both ventricles – more on the left, with mitral regurgitation. Prognosis is related to the severity of dysfunction. Significant cardiomegaly, low cardiac output and overt cardiac failure give a poor prognosis. There are many causes, including anomalies of the left coronary artery, arrhythmias, viral, protozoal and fungal myocarditis, anthracycline drugs, mucopolysaccharidosis, fatty acid oxidation defects, lipidosis, sialic acid storage disease, carnitine deficiency, amino acidaemia, muscular dystrophy, myopathies, Friedreich's ataxia, and some chromosomal abnormalities. Diuretics and digoxin will help initially, but adding captopril may be of value. Cardiac transplantation should be considered early.

Case 72

Answers: (a) 3
       (b) 3

Caudothalamic cyst

This is an incidental finding, and has no long-term complications. It usually disappears within the first 3–6 months of life. Follow-up scans at ages 3 and 6 months are required.

Case 73

Answers: (a) 1, 2, 5, 7, 8
       (b) 3

Smith–Lemli–Opitz syndrome

This is characterized by failure to thrive, short stature, ptosis, broad nasal bridge, upturned nose, micrognathia and microcephaly. Hypospadias, cryptorchidism, syndactyly of the 2nd and 3rd toes, low-set ears and simian creases are other features, although they are not always present. The child will be mentally retarded and developmentally delayed and will show marked hypotonia. Mortality is high in the first year of life. Abnormal gyration and cerebellar hypoplasia are common. The plasma cholesterol level is very low while the 7-dehydrocholesterol level is raised. Survival correlates with cholesterol plasma level: the higher the cholesterol, the greater is the chance of survival. A high-cholesterol regimen will normalize the level, but will not be clinically effective.

Case 74

Answers: (a) I
(b) 2, 4

Non-accidental injury

The spiral fracture seen on the X-ray of the left humerus should prompt suspicion of non-accidental injury. Such a fracture is likely to have been incurred through a twisting injury. Osteogenesis imperfecta (OI) predisposes to easy fracturing. However, there is no evidence of osteopaenia seen on the X-ray. OI can be ruled out by taking an accurate family history, enquiring specifically about easy fracturing, the presence of blue sclera, and hearing and dental problems. A skeletal survey should rule out the presence of other old or recent fractures and the presence of Wormian bones on skull X-ray. Skeletal surveys should include all parts of the skeleton (including fingers and toes). These should be reviewed and reported jointly by the most senior paediatrician and radiologist available. A small metaphyseal abnormality seen on the left leg X-ray suggestive of 'bucket handle' traction injury may easily be missed.

Case 75

Answers: (a) 4
(b) 4

Chest asymmetry

In newborns this can be pectus excavatum, pectus carinatum or just asymmetry. It usually has no effect on lung function, and babies and toddlers will develop normally. As they grow up, it become less obvious. Poland's syndrome is usually associated with absence of the pectoralis major and is associated with restricted movement of the affected arm. Harrison's sulcus is an indication of chronic lung diseases in older children.

Case 76

A term baby (who does not appear dysmorphic) chokes on feeding, and appears to be a mouth-breather.

What is the diagnosis?

1. Duplex renal system
2. Ureterorectal fistula
3. Tracheo-esophageal fistula
4. Left main bronchus obstruction
5. Left choanal atresia
6. Vaginal septal membrane
7. Double oesophageal channel

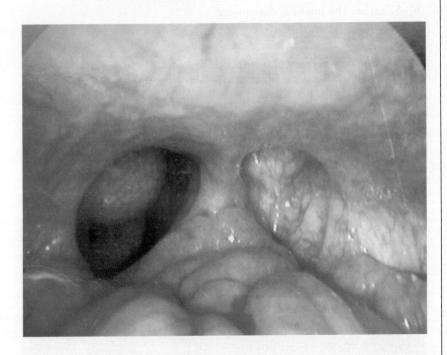

Case 77

In this 5-month-old girl cranial tomography was performed as part of an investigation of failure to thrive, poor head control and borderline large head. She is one of identical twins with no neonatal problems. There are no other dysmorphic features and all blood tests were reported as normal, including FBC, U&E, TFT, sweat test, Igs, amino acids, gases, lactate, blood sugar, chromosomes, TORCH screen, and urine organic acids and serum isotransferrin.

(a) **What are the three abnormalities seen here?**

    1. Bilateral dilated ventricles
    2. Cerebellar atrophy
    3. Right intraventricular haemorrhage
    4. Right ventricular mass
    5. Midline shift to left
    6. Cerebral oedema

(b) **What are the possible diagnoses?**

    1. Right intraventricular haemorrhages
    2. Right intraventricular cyst
    3. Right intraventricular astrocytoma
    4. Right intraventricular choroid plexus papilloma

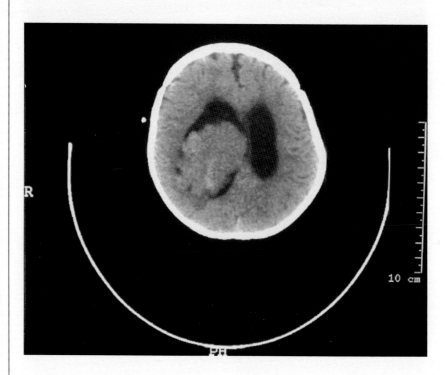

Case 78

This postmortem specimen slide is from a 6-month-old child who died of renal failure.

(a) What are the two abnormalities on this slide?

1. Bilateral polycystic disease
2. Bilateral renal scarring
3. Dilated right ureter
4. Urinary bladder mass
5. Scarred right kidney

(b) What is the diagnosis?

1. Reflux nephropathy
2. Bilateral hydronephrosis
3. Vesico-ureteric reflux
4. Bilateral polycystic renal disease
5. Posterior urethral valve obstruction

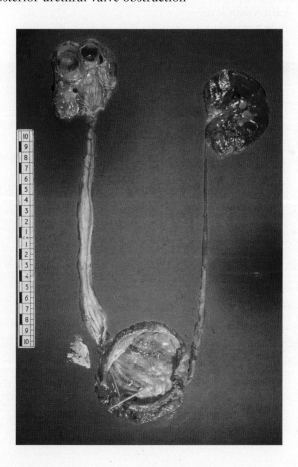

Case 79

A 2-week-old baby presents with a history of tachypnoea and not feeding very well. The radiologist reported the X-ray as abnormal with marked hyperinflation and no consolidation or air leaks.

(a) **What is the diagnosis?**

  1. Right middle lobe collapse
  2. Raised diaphragm on right
  3. Interstitial pneumonitis
  4. Congenital lobar emphysema
  5. Cystic fibrosis

(b) **What test would establish the diagnosis?**

  1. Immunoglobulin levels
  2. IgG subclass
  3. DNA linkage study for cystic fibrosis
  4. Echocardiography
  5. α_1-Antitrypsin level
  6. CT lung scan

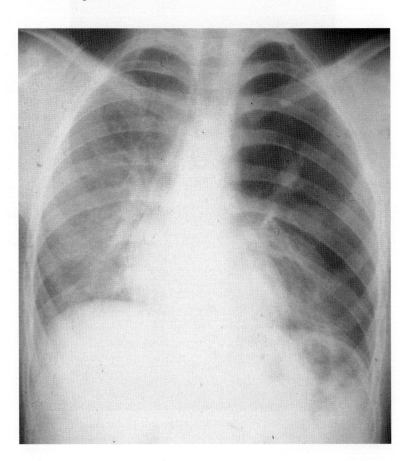

Case 80

This is a CT brain scan performed on a 9-month-old baby girl with a history of lethargy, vomiting, poor feeding and a single brief seizure. The baby was very irritable. The fontanel was full and tense. The temperature was 38.5°C; the CRP was 110 mmol/l and the coagulation screen was normal.

(a) **What is the diagnosis?**

   1. External hydrocephalus
   2. Bilateral frontal lobe atrophy
   3. Bilateral subdural effusion
   4. Generalized brain atrophy
   5. Craniosynostosis

(b) **What are the possible three causes in order?**

   1. Post bacterial meningitis
   2. Post trauma
   3. Non-accidental injury
   4. Congenital
   5. Metabolic disorders
   6. Post hypoxic ischemic encephalopathy
   7. Post viral meningitis

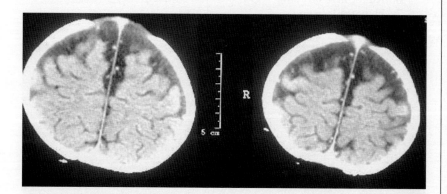

Case 81

A 4-year-old boy presented with shortness of breath, which was worse on lying down over the preceding 3 days. His liver and spleen were enlarged. He said that he had had a rash 2 days before, which had now disappeared. The blood film was reported as normal, with slightly low haemoglobin and raised ALT.

(a) **What are the two abnormalities on this X-ray?**

1. Right upper lobe collapse
2. Right upper lobe consolidation
3. Right upper lobe mass
4. Mediastinal mass
5. Hyperinflated lungs
6. Right middle lobe consolidation
7. Trachea shifted to left

(b) **What is the likely diagnosis?**

1. Pulmonary tuberculosis
2. Thymoma
3. Lymphoma
4. Acute lymphoblastic leukaemia
5. Infectious mononucleosis
6. Rhabdmyosarcoma
7. Hepatoblastoma

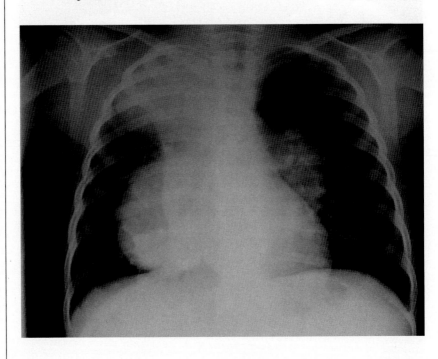

Case 82

A 4-month-old infant presented with swelling of the left side of the abdomen. Ultrasound showed a cystic lesion not communicating with any internal organs. The fluid is clear. There is no musculature involvement. The child is not in discomfort, but suffers from swollen limbs as well from time to time. Doppler ultrasound for vessels in the lower and upper limbs showed normal blood flow. Biopsy from the lump showed no evidence of any tumour cells and only bundles of lymphoid tissue.

What is the most likely diagnosis?

1. Lymphoma
2. Cystic hygroma
3. Lipoma
4. Rhabdomyosarcoma
5. Cavernous haemangioma
6. Stoma

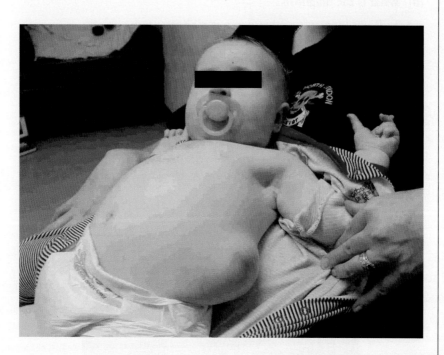

Case 83

This a chest X-ray of a 5-month-old girl with a history of tachypnoea from birth, cough and an abnormal shape of the chest. She has not been able to sleep over the last 2 days, with frequent cough and choking-like episodes from time to time. Her blood gas shows compensated respiratory acidosis; there is a normal eosinophil count and normal sweat and Heaf tests.

(a) **What are two abnormalities on this chest X-ray?**

1. Hyperinflated lungs
2. Mediastinum shifted to the right
3. Stomach on right side
4. Right lower lobe collapse
5. Right lower chest quadrant mass
6. Right lower lobe consolidation

(b) **What is the diagnosis?**

1. Right lung cystic adenomatous malformation
2. Right lower lobe collapse
3. Right diaphragmatic hernia
4. Right lower lobe arteriovenous malformation
5. Lymphoma

(c) **What other one investigation would you perform?**

1. Blood film
2. Bone marrow aspirate
3. Chest CT scan
4. Ventilation–perfusion scan
5. Lung function test
6. Lateral chest X-ray
7. Pulmonary venography
8. Barium swallow
9. Upper GIT endoscopy

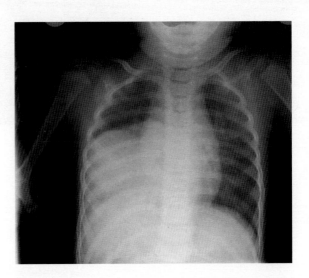

Case 84

A 3-month-old baby with a skin blemish over the leg:

What is the diagnosis?

1. Scarring following a cigarette burn
2. Dimple
3. Scarring from amniotic bands
4. Cavernous haemangioma
5. Absent radius
6. Keloid

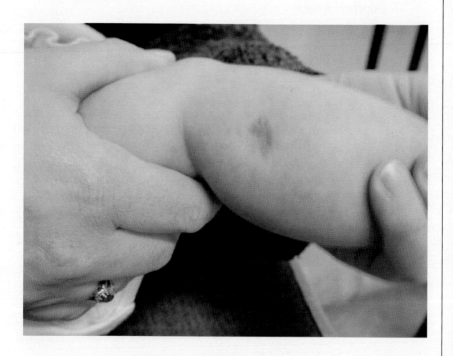

Case 85

This baby was stillborn at 33 weeks of gestation. The mother was 32 years old and this was her first baby. There were no other concerns during pregnancy and no previous miscarriages.

(a) **What are the abnormalities on these two photographs?**

1. Low-set ears
2. Long narrow head
3. Micrognathia
4. Narrow sloping palpebral fissure
5. Hypoplastic nails
6. Short nose
7. Short neck
8. Brachycephaly

(b) **What is the diagnosis?**

1. Patau's syndrome
2. Zellweger's syndrome
3. Edwards' syndrome
4. Down's syndrome
5. Cri-du-chat syndrome
6. Cornelia de Lange syndrome

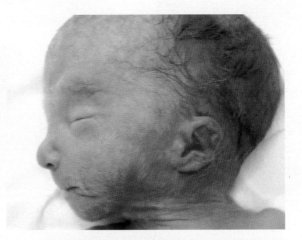

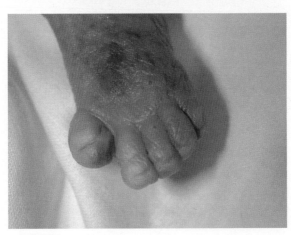

Case 86

A 3-year-old child presented to paediatric A&E with this rash. His mother described the rash as changing every hour, sometimes becoming dark blue and itchy. He is on ampicillin for a sore throat and tonsillitis. A throat swab grew β-haemolytic streptococci.

(a) **What is the diagnosis?**

1. Urticaria
2. Erythema multiforme
3. Vasculitis
4. Burns
5. Anaphylactic reaction

(b) **Name three possible causes**

1. Ampicillin
2. Exposure to allergen
3. Streptococcal throat infection
4. Herpes simplex infection
5. *Mycoplasma* pneumonia

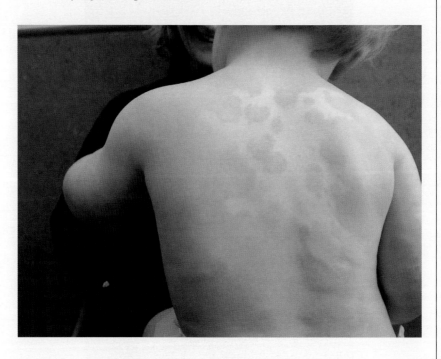

Case 87

Both of these babies are 1 day old. The baby in (i) was born vaginally. The father of this baby has a similar problem. The baby in (ii) was born by ELSCS with forceps assistance.

(a) **What are the diagnoses?**

    1. Left lower motor neurone 7th nerve palsy
    2. Bilateral 7th nerve palsy
    3. Right lower motor neurone 7th nerve palsy
    4. Right upper motor neurone 7th nerve palsy
    5. Left upper motor neurone 7th nerve palsy

(b) **Can any further test be performed?**

    1. Cranial MRI scan   **4.** Electromyography
    2. Cranial ultrasound   **5.** None
    3. 7th nerve conduction study

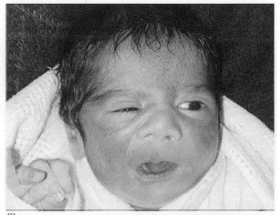

(i)

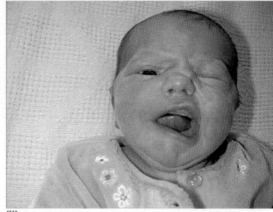

(ii)

Case 88

This is a chest X-ray of a 3-day-old full-term baby with a history of dusky episodes. The oxygen saturation is 90% in air and there is a soft ejection systolic murmur on the pulmonary area. There are no dysmorphic features and the baby is feeding very well. Chromosomes are reported as normal on karyotyping.

(a) **What are the two abnormalities on this chest X-ray?**

 1. Hyperinflated lungs
 2. Boot-shaped heart
 3. Stomach on right side
 4. Wide mediastinum
 5. Oligaemic lung fields
 6. Prominent pulmonary vessels

(b) **What is the possible diagnosis?**

 1. Upper airway obstruction
 2. Lower airway obstruction
 3. Tetralogy of Fallot
 4. Critical pulmonary stenosis
 5. Left ventricular hypoplastic syndrome
 6. Tracheo-oesophageal fistula

(c) **What is another test to confirm the diagnosis?**

 1. Chest CT
 2. Chest ultrasound
 3. Cardiac catheterization
 4. Echocardiography
 5. Fluorescence in situ hybridization (FISH) study for chromosome 22 deletion
 6. Bronchsocopy
 7. Ventilation–perfusion scan

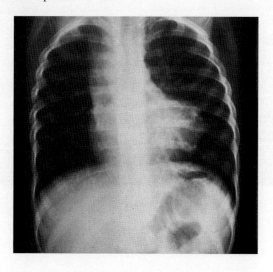

Case 89

This is an angiogram from a 2-year-old child presenting with a history of left-side hemiplegia, drowsiness and lethargy. His CT with enhancement shows an area of low density on the right parietotemporal area.

(a) **What is the diagnosis?**

1. Sturge–Weber syndrome
2. Vein of Galen malformation
3. Middle cerebral artery infarct
4. Plexiform papilloma
5. Intraventricular tumour

(b) **What are the possible complications?**

1. External hydrocephalus
2. Rupture
3. Heart failure
4. Mental retardation
5. Calcification of central grey matter
6. Early neonatal death

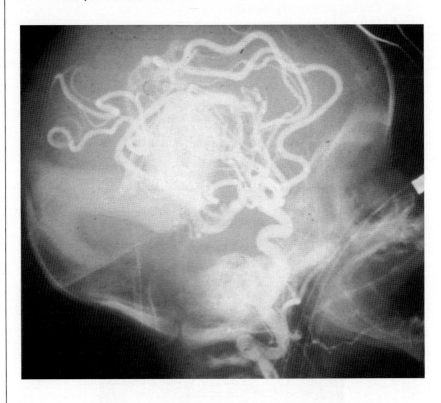

Case 90

This child was born with buphthalmus and found to be blind on the left side. His cranial MRI was normal and VEP was also normal. There was atrophy of the left optic nerve. The TORCH screen was normal. There were no birthmarks and no other abnormalities on systemic and general examination.

(a) **What single test would you like to ask the ophthalmologist to perform?**

    1. Fundoscopic examination
    2. Slit-lamp examination
    3. Measuring intraocular pressure
    4. Visual field
    5. Visual equity
    6. Nothing

(b) **What is the diagnosis?**

    1. Congenital cataract
    2. Congenital glaucoma
    3. Osteogenesis imperfecta
    4. Left iris coloboma
    5. Left corneal opacities
    6. Post-chickenpox corneal damage

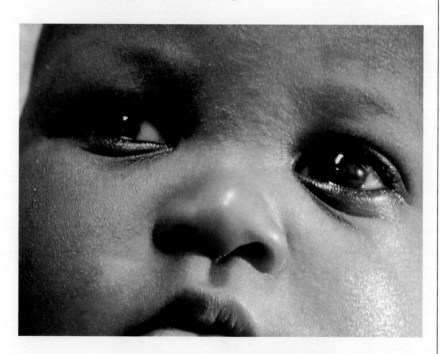

Case 91

This is a 1-day-old baby born by ELSCS. The parents were advised to terminate the pregnancy as everyone involved thought that this could be a variant of anencephaly.

(a) **What is the diagnosis?**

1. Encephalohaematoma
2. Haemangioma
3. Encephalocoele
4. Cystic hygroma
5. Anencephaly

(b) **What further test can be performed?**

1. Cranial ultrasound
2. Cranial CT
3. Cranial MRI scan
4. Cranial Doppler
5. Arterial angiography

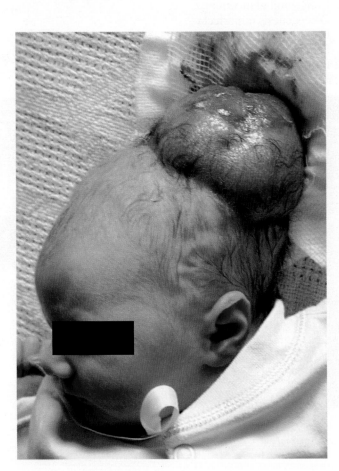

Case 92

This was the first baby for a couple from Albania. An antenatal scan at 22 weeks was normal.

(a) **What is the diagnosis?**

1. Congenital ichthyosis
2. Harlequin baby syndrome
3. Collodion baby syndrome

(b) **What is the inheritance?**

1. Autosomal recessive
2. Autosomal dominant
3. X-linked recessive
4. X-linked dominant
5. Sporadic
6. Multifactorial

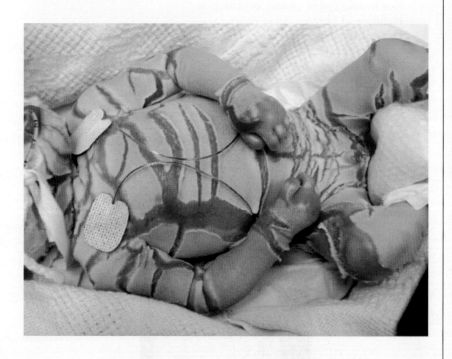

Case 93

This 9-year-old boy has suffered from asthma since the age of 2 years. He is on budesonide 600mg twice a day via an inhaler, salbutamol PRN and salmeterol 25mg twice a day and requires 6–8 courses of 3 days' oral prednisolone of 2mg/kg every year.

(a) **What is the abnormality?**

1. Pectus excavatum
2. Harrison's sulcus
3. Pectus carinatum
4. Pigeon chest wall
5. Poland's syndrome

(b) **What is the possible cause?**

1. Congenital
2. Chronic lower airway obstruction
3. Chronic upper airway obstruction
4. Bilateral phrenic nerve palsy
5. Bone dysplasia
6. Osteoporosis
7. Generalized osteomalacia

(c) **What routine test can be performed on him?**

1. Annual chest X-ray
2. Annual chest CT
3. Annual lung function test
4. Annual chest fluoroscopy
5. Annual bronchoscopy
6. Nothing

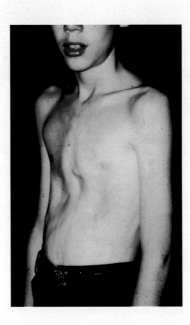

Case 94

This 4-year-old boy presented with a rash around and inside his mouth. He was admitted and treated for this, but 2 days later developed right-side hemiplegia with right-side 7th nerve involvement.

(a) **What is the diagnosis from the photograph?**

    1. Vasculitis
    2. Lip haemangioma
    3. Herpes gingivostomatitis
    4. Buccal fungal infection
    5. Non-accidental injury
    6. Angio-oedema
    7. Impetigo

(b) **What is the abnormality on the MRI scan?**

    1. Bilateral increase in white matter signals (occipital and temporal)
    2. Left occipital lobe infarct
    3. Left temporal lobe infarct
    4. Generalized cerebral oedema
    5. None

(c) **What is the diagnosis from the MRI and clinical history?**

    1. Herpes encephalitis
    2. Herpes myeloencephalitis
    3. Acute demyelinating encephalomyelitis
    4. Stroke
    5. Acute cerebritis

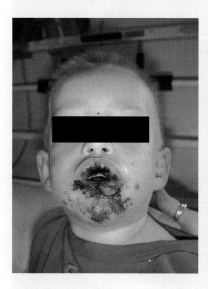
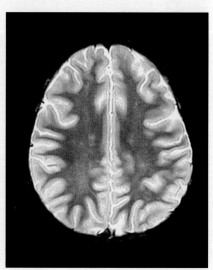

Case 95

A CT brain scan was performed on a 3-month-old infant with rapidly increasing head circumference.

(a) **What is the diagnosis?**

1. Non-communicating hydrocephalus
2. Communicating hydrocephalus
3. Posterior fossa tumour
4. Post-haemorrhagic hydrocephalus with bilateral resolving IVH

(b) **What are the possible causes?**

1. Aqueduct stenosis
2. Giant cell astrocytoma
3. Chiari malformation
4. Dandy–Walker cyst
5. Post-haemorrhagic
6. Craniopharyngioma
7. Toxoplasmosis
8. Meningitis
9. Hamartoma

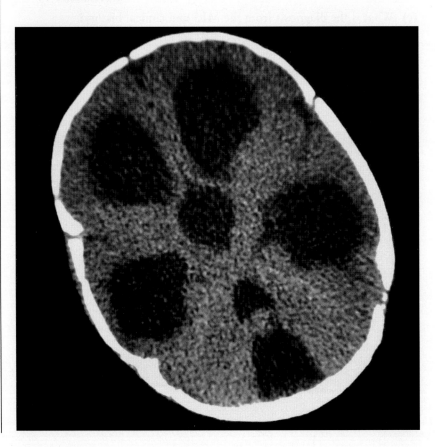

Case 96

This infant's penis was noted to have an unusual appearance:

What is the diagnosis?

1. Glandular hypospadias
2. Epispadias
3. Congenital adrenal hypoplasia
4. Volcano penis
5. Normal penis

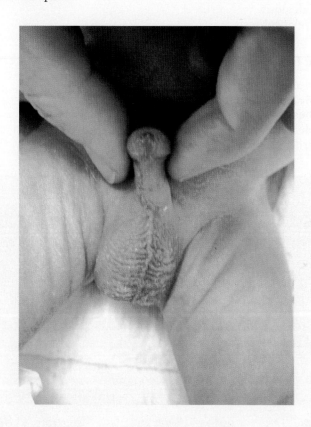

Case 97

An 8-week-old male infant born preterm at 26 weeks' gestation after a pregnany complicated by severe polyhydramnios fails to gain weight in the NICU. He has episodes of hyponatraemia and hypokalaemia. He undergoes a renal ultrasound scan.

(a) **What does the scan show?**

1. Dilated renal pelves
2. Bright corticomedullary junction
3. Calcinosis
4. Pyelonephrosis
5. Cystic-dysplastic disease

(b) **What further tests would you perform?**

1. Measure urinary calcium
2. Measure plasm rennin and aldosterone
3. Measure plasma 17α-hydroxyprogesterone
4. Measure plasma bicarbonate
5. Urine culture

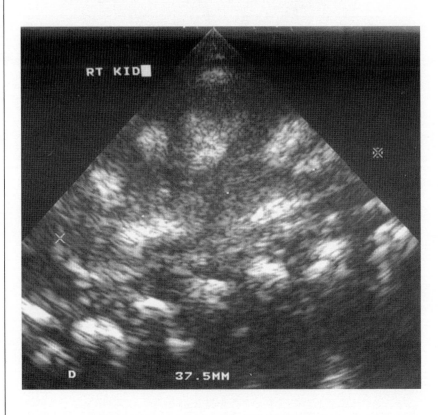

Case 98

This 3-month-old infant presented with lethargy and vomiting, and kept drawing his legs up to his chest. Extending his legs made him cry. He had not opened his bowels for the preceding 18 hours; his last feed was given 6 hours before and he vomited all of it.

What is the diagnosis from this abdominal X-ray?

1. Hirschsprung's disease
2. Intestinal malrotation
3. Paralytic ileus
4. Necrotizing enterocolitis
5. Obstructed right inguinal hernia
6. Obstructed left inguinal hernia
7. Intussusception
8. Volvulus
9. Intestinal obstruction due to abdominal mass

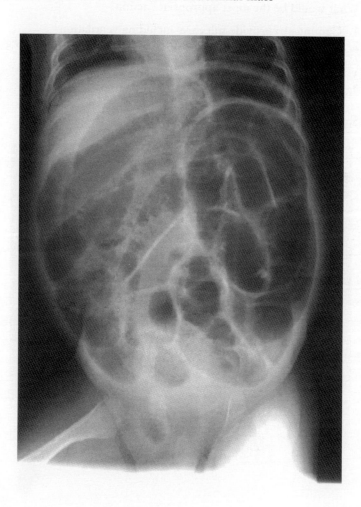

Case 99

A 1-week-old 31-week-gestation infant has a prolonged apnoeic attack requiring intubation and ventilation. Two days after the episode a cranial ultrasound scan is performed (i).

(a) **What abnormality does this scan demonstrate?**

   1. Bilateral intraventricular haemorrhages
   2. Normal appearances
   3. Bilateral subdural haemorrhages
   4. Unilateral cerebral oedema
   5. Ventriculitis

One week later the infant remains ventilated and is noted to have fixed dilated pupils with no spontaneous movement. A repeat cranial ultrasound scan is performed (ii). Discussions take place with all concerned (staff and family) on the future management.

(b) **What would be the most appropriate action?**

   1. Continue to provide full care, including ventilation
   2. Extubate the infant and withdraw all care, including feeding and fluids
   3. Extubate but continue to provide milk and fluids
   4. Refer to neurosurgeon for second-opinion reference ventricular shunt
   5. Extubate and administer morphine

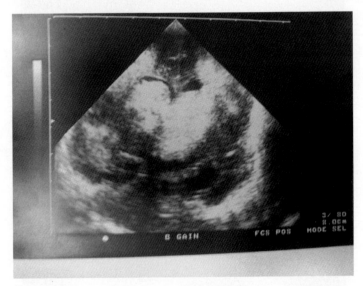

(i)

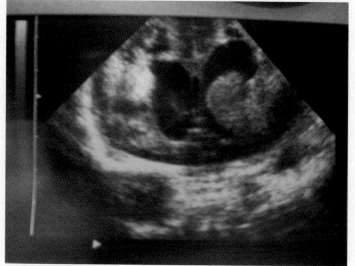

(ii)

Case 100

This is an 8-day-old boy, born at term. On day 2 he developed jaundice and his total bilirubin was 220 mmol/l. This was repeated on several occasions and he did not require phototherapy. He was slow feeding, and by day 5 his feeding became more problematic and he developed a fever. The scrotum became red and swollen. Blood culture was sent, as well as CRP, ESR and MSU.

(a) **What is the diagnoses?**

1. Torsion right testis
2. Cellulitis
3. Infected hydrocoele
4. Femoral vein thrombosis
5. Infected cavernous haemangioma
6. Allergic reaction to nappies

(b) **What other investigation is needed?**

1. Scrotal ultrasound
2. Abdominal ultrasound
3. Venography of left leg
4. Doppler ultrasound of left leg
5. MRI scan of left leg
6. Surgical exploration of the scrotum

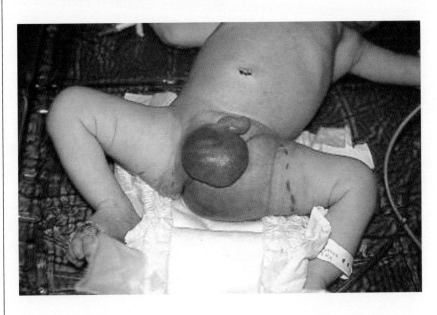

Case 76

Answer: 5

Choanal atresia

This is due to failure of breakdown of the nasobuccal membrane, which normally occurs at 6 weeks of gestation. It is usually unilateral, and 50% are associated with the CHARGE syndrome. If bilateral, it is dangerous and emergency management is required. Some patients can mouth-breath but have difficulties in feeding. The diagnosis can be made on the basis of suspicion and inability to pass a catheter along the nose. Establishing an airway is important before corrective surgery. A CT scan is required to determine the atresia before corrective surgery, and nasal endoscopy will also help. It is important to rule out other associations with this abnormality.

Case 77

Answers: (a) 1, 4, 5
      (b) 4

Choroid plexus papilloma

This is usually a benign tumour; it constitutes about 3% of childhood intracranial neoplasms. It arises from the epithelium of the choroid plexus. It is more common in infancy than in older children. Hydrocephalus is the usual manifestation in infancy, and is usually rapidly evolving and accompanied by papilloedema. The hydrocephalus is due to increased CSF production and is a communicating hydrocephalus. Excision is the treatment of choice; a shunt is sometimes required. The prognosis is very good.

Case 78

Answers: (a) 1, 3
(b) 4

Renal cystic diseases

Renal cysts are relatively common lesions in adults. They may be single or multiple, cortical or medullary, sporadic or familial. There are various inherited forms; they can be associated with tuberous sclerosis, neurofibromatosis type 1, cerebrohepatorenal (Zellweger's) syndrome, Von Hippel–Lindau syndrome and trisomy 13 syndrome. Infantile autosomal recessive polycystic kidney disease can be diagnosed antenatally with enlarged kidneys and is hyperechoic on ultrasound. The cysts are fusiform and radially oriented. The liver is always fibrosed if biopsied. If the child has sufficient lung function, it will survive but renal failure will occur and renal transplant must be considered very early. The adult type is autosomally inherited and may cause renal failure. Familial juvenile nephronophthisis is inherited in an autosomal recessive manner. It usually presents at age 8–10 years with failure to grow, anaemia, polyuria and polydipsia. Chronic renal failure will occur. Renal transplant will be required. Medullary cystic diseases are similar to familial juvenile nephronophthisis but present in adult life.

Case 79

Answers: (a) 4
(b) 6

Congenital lobar emphysema

This uncommon condition is due to bronchial obstruction or deficiency of bronchial cartilage. It is characterized by overinflation of one or more lobes. It is usually unilateral and the left upper and right middle lobe are the most commonly affected. Presentation can be with respiratory distress soon after birth and wheezes. CT lung scan confirms the diagnosis. Bronchoscopy is occasionally performed if a removable cause of bronchial obstruction is found. In 30% of cases it is associated with congenital heart defects. Sometimes surgical excision of the affected lobe is required, but conservative management is often effective.

Case 80

Answers: (a) 3

(b) 1, 2, 3

Post bacterial meningitis subdural effusion

It is well recognized that following *Haemophilus influenzae* meningitis, subdural effusion is common, but this type of meningitis is hardly evet seen in Western Europe and America since the introduction of the HiB vaccine in the early 1990s. The fluid is usually high in albumin but with no blood. Although the subdural effusion is very common, no action is needed as it will resolve spontaneously. It is also associated with pneumococcal bacterial meningitis, but is then less dramatic and hardly causes problems. A CT scan is helpful, and a persistent high temperature and neurological deficit may indicate the presence of effusion in children with bacterial meningitis. Seizures can be associated with children who have effusion in the acute phase, but there is no longer-term increase in the incidence of seizures in children with postbacterial meningitis subdural effusions. No invasive therapy needed in any of these cases.

Case 81

Answers: (a) 3, 4, 7

(b) 3

Lymphoblastic lymphoma

This presents with a mediastinal mass in 70% of patients. There can be pleural effusion or superior vena caval obstruction, or dysphagia and dyspnoea. The lymphadenopathy is confined to the neck and axilla. Gross hepatosplenomegaly is common with CNS involvement. There is an increase in more mature T lymphocytes. Intensive multiagent chemotherapy gives a 60–80% survival rate.

Case 82

Answer: 2

Cystic hygroma

This commonly arises in the neck as a fluid-filled lesion of lymphatic origin. It can found anywhere there is lymphatic drainage, including axilla, abdominal wall and trunk. It may present at birth or within the first 2 years of life. Surgical excision should be performed early. Aspiration of the cysts and injection of the antitumour agent OK432 is a new treatment.

Case 83

Answers: (a) 4, 5

  (b) 3

  (c) 3

Diaphragmatic hernia

This can be congenital or acquired. There are three types. The Bochdalek type is a posterolateral defect. Hernia through the foramen of Morgagni is less common in neonates. It is a retrosternal defect on the right or left of the midline. The third type is an oesophageal hiatus hernia. Some are detected antenatally, but the majority present with respiratory distress with tachypnoea, dyspnoea and sometimes cyanosis. This can be immediately or within the first few hours after birth. The presentation can be late, especially on the right side. The later the presentation, the better the prognosis. There is a scaphoid abdomen, a shift of the mediastinum, and bowel sounds in the chest or a marked reduced air entry on the right side if it is a right diaphragmatic hernia. An ultrasound scan will help the initial diagnosis, but chest CT is the diagnostic procedure and will help to plan surgery. Surgery should be performed immediately. If presented at birth, the baby should be intubated and ventilated, with correction of acidosis. Pulmonary vascular resistance should be controlled and pCO_2 kept < 5.3 kPa and ventilatory index < 1000. Delaying surgery and giving the lungs a chance to grow is another option that some centres have adopted with encouraging results.

Case 84

Answer: 2

Dimple

This is usually congenital as a result of pressure or an amniotic band. The commonest site is the sacral region, where it is sometimes connected with the spinal canal. If a dimple is seen on the lumbosacral region during the baby check, an attempt should be made to see the bottom of the dimple and if it is not seen, an ultrasound scan should be performed. A blind tract needs no further management. Sacro-coccygeal dimples and pits do not need to be probed or investigated.

Case 85

Answers: (a) 1, 2, 3, 4, 5
  (b) 3

Edwards' syndrome (trisomy 18)

There is often polyhydramnios with intrauterine growth retardation. The cranium is long and narrow with a prominent occipital. Low-set ears, micrognathia and sloping of the palpeberal fissure are other characteristic features. The hands are clenched with third and fourth fingers overlapping. The nails are hypoplastic and the feet show a rocker bottom appearance. Other anomalies include intestinal atresias, exomphalos, malabsorption, renal hypoplasia, congenital heart diseases, ocular abnormalities and neural tube defects. Trisomy 18 is usually not compatible with life; the majority are stillbirths and few can survive for more than 12 months.

Case 86

Answers: (a) 2
  (b) 1, 4, 5

Erythema multiforme

These are the three most common causes. Vasculitis, which is predominantly lymphocytic, is prominent on histological examination. The role of the immune complex system in this condition is still not known, but there is some evidence that intravascular IgM and C3 are associated with the vasculitis. A circular target lesion is the most common characteristic feature. This occurs mainly on the limbs, with a red periphery and blue centre. If it is bullous then the child will be ill and toxic (Stevens–Johnson syndrome). It usually disappears within 10 days, but may reappear where herpes simplex is the cause. The eyes can be affected. Treatment is usually aggressive and the use of steroids is not contraindicated.

Case 87

Answers: (a) (i) 5, (ii) 3
  (b) 5

Facial nerve palsy

This is usually congenital, but can be acquired as a result of trauma. The congenital form can involve just the 7th nerve and shows the usual upper motor neurone signs. It may be associated with others such as bilateral 6th nerve palsy and bilateral 7th nerve palsy (Möbius syndrome). If traumatic in orgin, it is usually of the lower motor neurone type; following forceps delivery, it is very rare, and recovery can be within a couple of weeks. The congenital form will not disappear, and cosmetic surgery and looking after the eyes are very important.

Case 88

Answers: (a) 2, 5

(b) 3

(c) 4

Tetralogy of Fallot

Babies with tetralogy of Fallot are not usually cyanosed at birth but become so with time. Intrauterine diagnosis is now possible. The majority of cases develop by the end of the first year of life. A diagnosis of ventricular septal defect or pulmonary stenosis can be made and tetralogy of Fallot can be missed. The occurrence of cyanotic attacks is another feature due to spasm of the pulmonary infundibular muscle leading to reduced pulmonary blood flow. They occur in the morning, or when the baby is crying, and are life-threatening. Children with pulmonary atresia and VSD will present after birth with cyanosis. Surgical repair is the definitive treatment, but this depends on the anatomy, the clinical symptoms and the experience and policy of the surgical team. Total correction can be done or the Blalock–Taussig operation (the subclavian artery is transected and anastomosed to the pulmonary artery) can be performed followed by total correction at 2–4 years of age.

Case 89

Answers: (a) 2

(b) 1, 2, 3, 4, 5, 6

Vein of Galen malformation

This is an arteriovenous malformation that results from abnormal communication between one or several cerebral arteries and the vein of Galen. The most common clinical manifestation is heart failure due to high flow through the malformation. It can cause progressive hydrocephalus as a result of increasing venous pressure or of compression of the sylvian aqueduct. Definitive diagnosis is by cranial tomography or MRI scan and by angiography. In neonates the prognosis is poor and many die from heart failure. The use of anticongestive and cardiotonic drugs will buy time for corrective surgery in most patients. When cardiac function is stabilized, corrective surgery can be performed by reduction of the flow through the fistula (best done at age 6 months). Alternatively, vaso-occlusive embolization of the feeding arteries by interventional radiology may be used.

Case 90

Answers: (a) 3

(b) 2

Congenital glaucoma (buphthalmus)

This is caused by a congenital anatomical anomaly in the angle of the anterior chamber that interferes with drainage of the aqueous humour. The anatomical defect is variable and present at birth, but the enlargement of the eye appears when the child is few months old (sometimes at age 1–3 years). There will be progressive enlargement of the eye, especially the anterior posterior diameter, due to an increase in intraocular pressure. The child will suffer from myopia and the cornea will become hazy due to oedema followed by rupture of Descemet's membrane and reddening of the eye, photophobia, and epiphora. The optic nerve head will become atrophic and cupped. In this case the damage to vision will be permanent if treatment is not applied immediately. Trabeculotomy is the treatment of choice. Secondary buphthalmus can be due to uveitis, ocular neoplasm, intraocular haemorrhage or trauma. Sturge–Weber syndrome can cause glaucoma.

Case 91

Answers: (a) 3

(b) 3

Encephalocoele

This a mesenchymal defect with herniation of the dura, cerebral or cerebellar tissue, or ventricles. It is associated with other abnormalities such as agenesis of the corpus callosum or abnormal gyration. It is more common than spina bifida. Worldwide, more than two-thirds of cases are posteriorly located, although in Asia anterior encephalocoele is more common. The bony defect can be any size. The prognosis for posterior encephalocoele is poor, with more than half of patients developing hydrocephalus. Anterior encephalocoele can be associated with other abnormalities such as coloboma or optic atrophy. The prognosis is much better than for posterior encephalocoele.

Case 92

Answers: (a) 2

(b) 1

Harlequin baby syndrome

This is recessively inherited, and various abnormalities of keratinization and epidermal lipid metabolism have been demonstrated. Usually the baby is covered with thick dark plates of scale with severe ectropian, deformed ears, and claw hands and feet. Most babies die as neonates and those who survive will develop a type of ichthyosis.

Case 93

Answers: (a) 2
         (b) 2
         (c) 3

Harrison's sulcus

This is usually an indication of chronic lung disease associated with lower airway obstruction: asthma, cystic fibrosis, chronic small-airway diseases and rickets. It is usually due to prolonged diaphragmatic traction.

Case 94

Answers: (a) 3
         (b) 1
         (c) 3

Acute disseminated encephalomyelitis (ADEM)

This usually follows upper respiratory tract infection or an exanthematous disease. It is usually associated with widespread CNS disturbances, with coma, drowsiness, seizures and multifocal neurological problems. The involvement of grey matter favours a diagnosis of ADEM rather than multiple sclerosis. The EEG will be abnormal with a slow background and spikes may be seen periodically. The CSF will show pleocytosis and a mild increase in protein. MRI will show an increased signal on T2-weighted images, predominantly involving the white matter. The spinal cord may also be involved. Treatment with steroids will help. There should be follow-up MRI scans for a couple of years as persistence of white matter changes may indicate multiple sclerosis.

Case 95

Answers: (a) 1
         (b) All

Non-communicating hydrocephalus

This is complete obstruction of the pathway of cerebrospinal fluid from the ventricles to the subarachnoid space, which can cause an increase in pressure and dilatation of all ventricles. It is the commonest form of hydrocephalus. The causes include aqueduct stenosis (due to infection or inherited in an X-linked manner), Chiari malformation, Dandy–Walker cyst, Klippel–Feil syndrome, mass lesions (e.g. abscess, haematoma or tumour), vein of Galen malformation and Warburg's syndrome. Non-communicating hydrocephalus if associated with aqueduct stenosis needs a ventriculoperitoneal shunt. This will increase the potential for normal development.

Case 96

Answer: 1

Hypospadias

This is one of the most common congenital abnormalities, occurring in 1 in 400 live male births. The meatus lies on the ventral part of the penile shaft or even scrotally or perineally. The penis is deficient in foreskin and is described as a 'hooded penis' (glandular). It is also associated with chordee, which is ventral flexion of the penis. Sometimes the meatus is narrow and causes back-pressure. The surgical correction is preferably done at school age, and no circumcision should be performed before this as the foreskin can be used for total correction.

Case 97

Answers: (a) 3
(b) 1, 2, 4

Bartter's syndrome

The renal ultrasound scan shows nephrocalcinosis. This finding together with the clinical history of severe polyhydramnios and poor ante- and postnatal growth raises the possible diagnosis of Bartter's syndrome. The electrolyte abnormalities are consistent with the diagnosis and are caused by a salt-losing tubulopathy, which can result in water loss. Metabolic alkalosis is often found and hypertension may occur as a result of secondary hyper-reninaemia and hyperaldersteronism. The syndrome is inherited in an autosomal recessive manner and is caused by one of several possible mutations in genes coding for sodium, potassium and chloride transport proteins. Treatment involves replacement of fluid and electrolyte losses plus the administration of indomethacin.

Case 98

Answer: 5

Inguinal hernia

The presence of a patent processus vaginalis if wide will produce a hernia and if narrow will produce a hydrocoele. A complete inguinal hernia results when the processus vaginalis is persistently wide open. Obliteration of the distal part results in a funicular hernia. It is more common on the right due to the later decent of the right testis. If found in girls, a chromosomal study should be performed. Clinical examination is important to differentiate between hydrocoele and inguinal hernia. It is possible to get above a hydrocoele but not above a hernia. Incarceration of an inguinal hernia implies irreducibility, which can lead to strangulation of the bowel. Before surgery, gentle reduction should be attempted; if the hernia is irreducible then emergency surgery is required (herniotomy). Even if reduction is possible, herniotomy should not be delayed (and preferably should be performed during the same admission).

Case 99

Answers: (a) 1

(b) 3

Bilateral intraventricular haemorrhages

The initial cerebral ultrasound scan shows bilateral intraventricular haemorrhages with probable extensive venous cerebral infarction (grade IV IVH). The follow-up scan shows evolution of the haemorrhage in association with ventricular dilatation and extensive bilateral cystic changes and cerebral damage. A subsequent MRI brain scan confirmed the extent of the damage.

The management of such infants is fraught with ethical and practical difficulties. The Royal College of Paediatrics and Child Health suggests the following situations where withholding or withdrawal of curative medical treatment might be considered (RCPCH. *Withholding or Withdrawing Life Sustaining Treatment in Children: A Framework for Practice*, 2nd ed. London: RCPCH, 2004):

1. The brain-dead child
2. The permanent vegetative state
3. The no-chance situation
4. The no-purpose situation
5. The unbearable situation.

The final decision to withdrawal life support must lie with the named consultant responsible for the infant. The decision should only be arrived at after agreement with the parents following close discussions on the reasons for withdrawal. It is in the interests of the named consultant to have a second consultant present (preferably not part of the treatment team) at the time of the discussion and for both consultants to sign their written opinions and decisions in the clinical notes. Other members of the care team, including nursing staff and middle-grade doctors, should also be included in discussions.

Case 100

Answers: (a) 2

(b) 1

Cellulitis

This is an acute bacterial infection affecting the subcutis and the dermis. The lesion is erythematous with purple or blue hue. It is warm and tender and has a poorly defined edge. Fever, tiredness, leucocytosis and lymphadenopathy usually present. Group A β-haemolytic streptococci are the organisms most commonly involved if the infection is associated with broken skin. Other organisms that can cause cellulitis are *Haemophilus influenzae*, *Streptococcus pneumoniae*, *Staphylococcus aureus* and *Pseudomonas aeruginosa*.

Case 101

This is a chest X-ray of 9-year-old boy who presented with a history of fever, malaise, cough and not feeling well over the last 2 days. He said that his throat was hurting as well as his legs. The white cell count was $17 \times 10^9/l$ with neutrophilia, CRP was 95 mg/l and there was reduced air entry on the right upper chest.

(a) What are the possible four organisms that can cause these changes?

1. *Pseudomonas aeruginosa*
2. *Escherichia coli*
3. *Pneumococcus pneumoniae*
4. *Klebsiella* spp.
5. *Staphylococcus aureus*
6. *Mycobacterium* spp.
7. *Mycoplasma* spp.

(b) What three further investigations would you perform?

1. Sputum analysis
2. Gastric lavage
3. Chest ultrasound
4. Bronchoscopy
5. CT lung scan

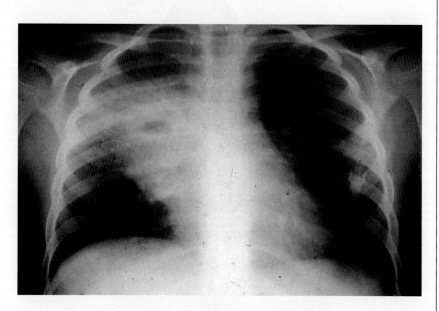

Case 102

This 15-month-old girl weighs only 7.2 kg and suffers from persistent cough and loose stools. She is neutropenic, with normal thyroid function test and normal immunoglobulins. Her father died from throat cancer 5 months ago. The sweat test is negative as is a DNA linkage study for ΔF_{508}.

(a) **What are your initial lines of investigation?**

1. Include metabolic screen
2. Do not include metabolic screen
3. Perform a head MRI scan
4. Do not perform a head MRI scan
5. Chromosome analysis
6. Coeliac screen
7. Upper and lower GIT endoscopy
8. Chest X-ray

(b) **What could this child have?**

1. Simple calorie problem
2. Chronic infection
3. Mother suffering from depression
4. Metabolic disorders
5. Child abuse
6. Nothing at all

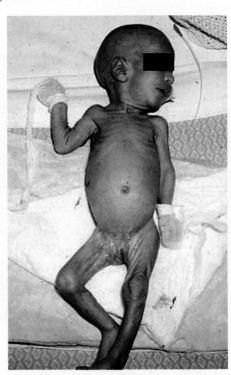

Case 103

This 3-year-old child had a 3-month history of abdominal pain.

(a) **What is the abnormality on this photograph?**

    1. None
    2. Bruises at 6 o'clock position
    3. Fissure at 7 o'clock position
    4. Old scar at 11 o'clock position
    5. Haemorrhoids

(b) **What are the possible causes?**

    1. Sexual abuse
    2. Accidental trauma
    3. Constipation
    4. Proctitis
    5. Crohn's disease

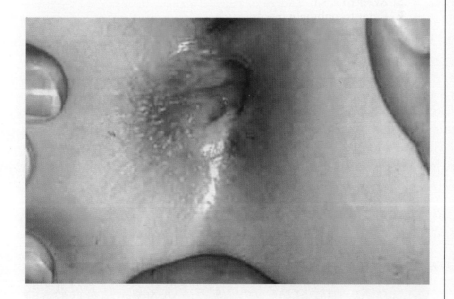

Case 104

This 14-year-old boy suffers from a swollen right eye and says that his vision has been blurred for the last 2 days. His headache is very severe and responds only to ibuprofen, which he has been taking over the last 2 weeks. There is no vomiting and there are no other problems. There is no history of trauma or other family illnesess.

(a) **What is the diagnosis from the CT scan?**

    1. Optic neuritis
    2. Pre-septal orbital cellulitis
    3. Septal orbital cellulitis
    4. Right maxillary sinusitis
    5. Zygomatic bone osteomyelitis

(b) **What is the best way to manage him?**

    1. Intravenous antibiotics
    2. Refer to ENT
    3. Refer to ophthalmologist
    4. No referral
    5. Cranial MRI scan

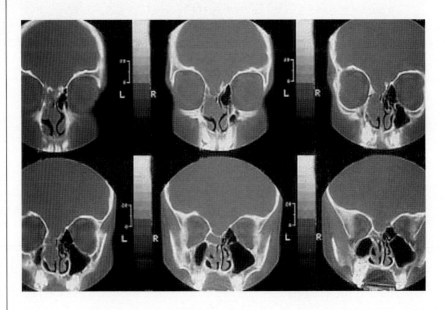

Case 105

An infant undergoes an MCUG after a urine infection.

(a) **What are the abnormalities on this MCUG?**

  1. None
  2. Bilateral vesico-ureteric reflux
  3. Complete duplex system on right side
  4. Partial duplex of the right kidney
  5. Ureterocoele
  6. Dilated ureter

(b) **What other tests might you perform?**

  1. Renal MRI scan
  2. DMSA scan
  3. Indirect cystogram: MAG3
  4. Functional urodynamic study
  5. IVU

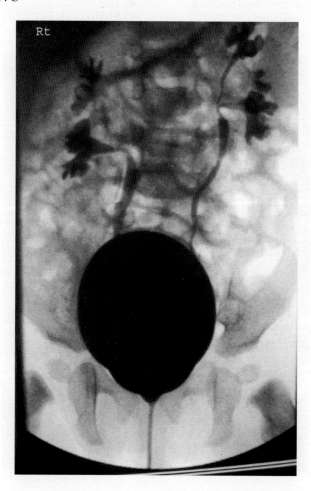

Case 106

An ex-preterm baby born at 26 weeks needed 7 days on ventilation and inotropic support for 3 days for low blood pressure. He subsequently did well and was sent home at the age of term plus 2 weeks. He presented to A&E with a history of generalized tonic/clonic seizures lasting 3 minutes, from which he recovered. His fontanelles were bulging but not tense. He was drowsy but interested in his feeding. He was admitted overnight and in the morning was found apparently lifeless; he was resuscitated and transferred to PICU.

(a) **What is the diagnosis from this CT scan?**

1. Bilateral subdural effusion	4. Intraventricular bleed
2. Generalized brain atrophy	5. Cerebral oedema
3. Severe hydrocephalus	

(b) **What could be the causes of this condition?**

1. Shaken baby syndrome	4. Unknown
2. Prematurity	5. Hydrocephalus
3. Birth trauma	

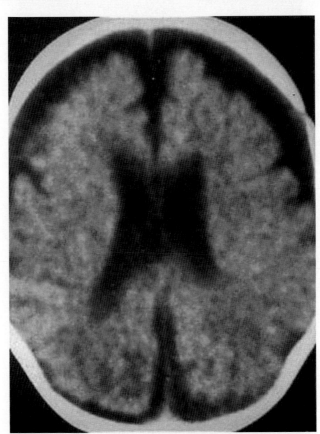

Case 107

This girl presented with a history of headache over the last 9 months and had missed a lot of school. Her mother was concerned about her weight, as she had gained 2 stones over the last 4 months. She also said that her concentration at school was not as good as before and on many occasions she had hit the left side of her head, which is why she had this X-ray taken. She said that she was no longer interested in school and wanted to leave.

(a) **What are the abnormalities on this skull X-ray?**

1. Widening of sutures
2. Fracture of occipital bone on right side
3. Fracture of the right orbital bone
4. Widening of pituitary fossa
5. 'Beaten copper' appearance of the skull
6. Osteomalacia of skull bones
7. Calcification of sella turcica of pituitary fossa

(b) **What other three investigations would you carry out?**

1. Bony window CT
2. AP skull X-ray
3. Cranial MRI scan
4. Renal ultrasound
5. LFT
6. PTH, Ca and phosphate levels
7. TFT, GH and cortisol levels
8. Serum and urine osmolality

(c) **What single bedside test would you perform?**

1. Urine analysis for proteins
2. Blood pressure
3. Visual fields
4. Visual acuity
5. Fog test

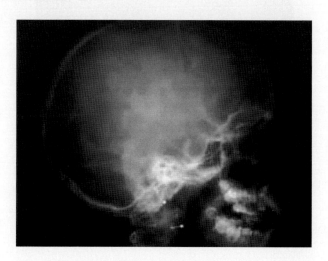

Case 108

This is an X-ray of a baby with pneumothorax.

What single procedure would you perform on this baby?

1. Insert an apical butterfly needle into the right 2nd intercostal space
2. Insert a midaxillary chest drain in the 4th right intercostal space
3. Put the child on 100% oxygen
4. Call for a consultant
5. Change endotracheal tube

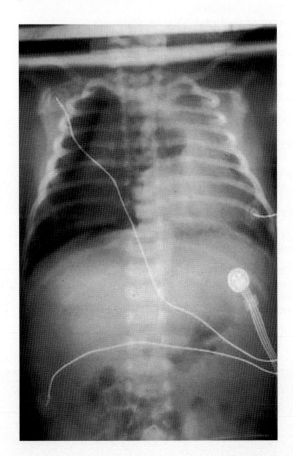

Case 109

This is a biopsy from the jejunum of a child with a history of poor weight gain and abdominal pain.

(a) **What are the abnormalities in (i) and (ii)?**

1. Lymphocytic infiltration
2. Absent of goblet cells
3. Total villous atrophy
4. No crypt formation
5. Normal tissue
6. Presence of cysts and oocytes

(b) **What is the diagnosis?**

1. Cow's milk protein intolerance
2. Giardiasis
3. Coeliac disease
4. IgA deficiency
5. Crohn's disease
6. Tropical sprue

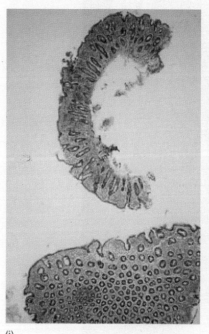

(i)

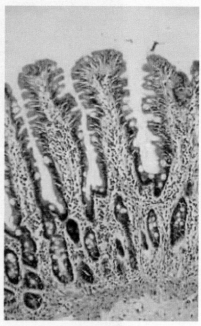

(ii)

Case 110

This is an X-ray of a 15-year-old girl with a long-standing history of painful joints.

(a) **What three abnormalities do you see on this film?**

    1. Osteopenia
    2. Osteoporosis
    3. Fused interphalangeal joints
    4. Fused metacarpal and carpal bones
    5. Calcification of terminal phalanges
    6. Dislocated interphalangeal joints
    7. Osler nodules

(b) **What are the possible diagnoses?**

    1. Juvenile chronic arthritis
    2. Psoriatic arthropathy
    3. Paget's disease
    4. SLE with arthropathy
    5. Renal osteopathy

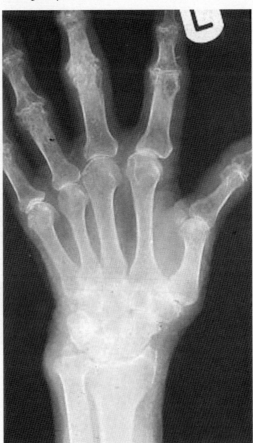

Case 111

This child suffers from recurrent hemiplegia and headaches.

(a) **What are the abnormalities on this angiogram?**

1. None
2. Multiple small arterial aneurysms
3. Puff of smoke appearance
4. Collateral arteries
5. Stenosis of large arteries

(b) **What is the diagnosis?**

1. Cerebral artery vasculitis
2. Cranial arteritis
3. Moya moya disease
4. Middle cerebral artery stenosis
5. Multiple aneurysm

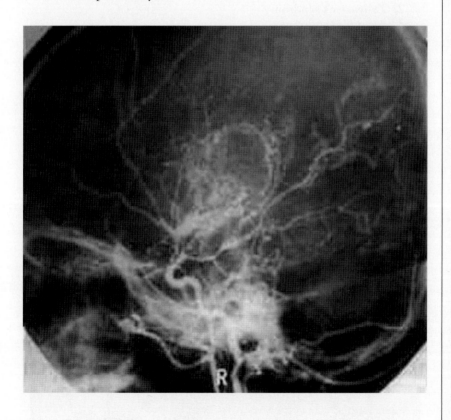

Case 112

This is cranial MRI (T1-weighted images) of a 6-month-old child with infantile spasms, hypsarrythmia, developmental delay and left micro-ophthalmia.

(a) **What are the abnormalities on this MRI?**

1. Bilateral large lateral ventricles
2. Generalized atrophy of the brain
3. Heterotopias, left frontal region
4. Periventricular heterotopias
5. Absent corpus callosum
6. Increased signals around the presylvian fissure
7. Polymicrogyria on the right frontal region

(b) **What is the diagnosis?**

1. Incontinentia pigmenti
2. Zellweger's syndrome
3. Aicardi's syndrome
4. West's syndrome
5. Patau's syndrome
6. Angelman's syndromes
7. Smith–Magenis syndrome

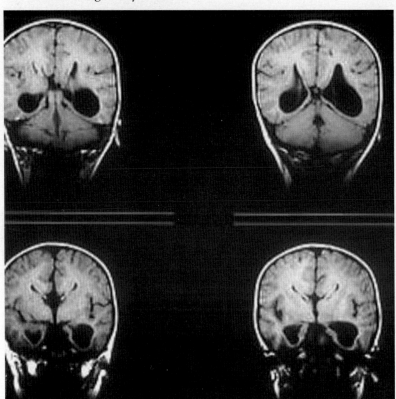

Case 113

This child was brought to hospital with swelling on the right side of her head. Her parents said that she had fallen after tumbling on the patio. This had happened 3 hours beforehand. The child looked very well otherwise.

(a) **What is the abnormality on this skull X-ray?**

1. None
2. Hydrocephalus
3. Craniosynostosis
4. Fracture of the right parietotemporal bone
5. Fracture of the left parietotemporal bone

(b) **How are you going to manage this child?**

1. Send her home with her parents
2. Refer to neurosurgeon
3. Refer to plastic surgeon
4. Refer to child protection team
5. Discuss with your consultant
6. Cranial tomography

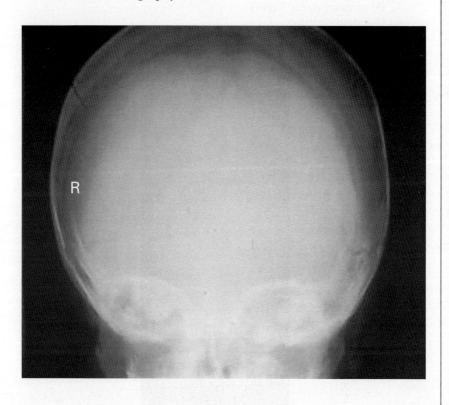

Case 114

This child was referred to the paediatrician because of frequent upper respiratory infections.

(a) **What are the abnormalities in (i)–(iii)?**

   1. None
   2. Otitis media
   3. Bulging tympanic membrane
   4. Perforated tympanic membrane
   5. Dull retracted tympanic membrane with fluid behind the membrane
   6. Foreign body in ear canal
   7. Otitis externa

(b) **How would you treat each of them?**

   1. Nothing
   2. Analgesia
   3. Antihistamine
   4. Oral antibiotics for 5 days
   5. IV antibiotics for 5 days
   6. Pseudoephedrine
   7. Referral to ENT surgeon
   8. Referral for hearing test in 2 months' time

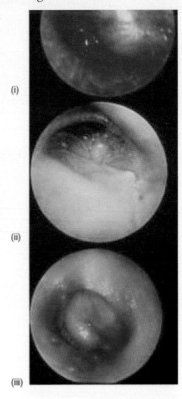

(i)

(ii)

(iii)

Case 115

This child was referred by social services as this mark was found while the child was crying. He had been seen a day earlier in A&E with abdominal pain. Blood had been taken and was reported as normal.

What is the diagnosis?

1. Adult bite mark
2. Child bite mark
3. Burn
4. Bruise
5. Site of venous access

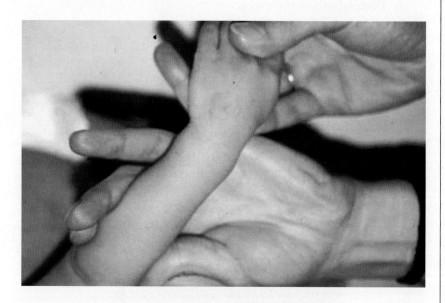

Case 116

This is a CT scan of a child presenting with infantile spasm, macrocephaly and stiffness in her lower limb. She responds well to vigabatrin and steroids.

(a) **What are the abnormalities on this CT scan?**

    1. Dilated bilateral ventricles
    2. Absence of corpus callosum
    3. Neuronal migration defect
    4. Smooth brain surfaces
    5. Periventricular calcification
    6. Bilateral subdural effusion

(b) **What is the diagnosis?**

    1. Hydrocephalus
    2. Brain atrophy secondary to HIE
    3. Lissencephaly
    4. Heterotopias
    5. Cortical dysplasia
    6. Tuberous sclerosis
    7. NF1
    8. Aicardi's syndrome

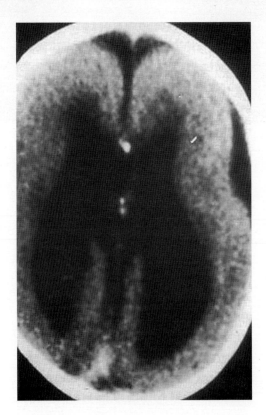

Case 117

This is a CT scan of a 13-year-old boy found unconcious at the side of the road.

(a) **What are the abnormalities on this scan?**

1. Right parietotemporal subdural collection
2. Cerebral oedema
3. Right frontal lobe haemorrhage
4. Skull fracture (left parietotemporal bone)
5. Midline shift to left
6. Midline shift to right
7. Right parietotemporal extradural collection

(b) **What are the steps of immediate management?**

1. Repeat CT scan after 2 hours
2. Call the anaesthetist
3. Immediate drainage of fluid
4. Give mannitol
5. Urgent referral to neurosurgeon
6. Admit to observation ward
7. Give phenobarbital
8. Give IV antibiotics
9. Perform cranial MRI
10. Insert central line

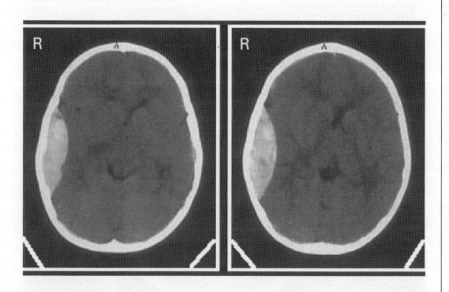

Case 118

This 12-year-old girl presented to A&E with severe headaches over the preceding 2 hours. She was conscious and able to walk without problems. While she was in A&E, she lost consciousness and her GCS dropped to 7. An anaesthetist was called and while he was intubating her, her pupils became dilated and unreactive. Her head was tipped back hard at the time. It was returned to the upright position and her pupils reacted to light again. She was intubated with her head in the upright position (30°).

(a) **What are the abnormalities on this contrast CT scan?**

1. Cerebral oedema
2. Posterior fossa mass
3. Extradural collection on left frontal region
4. Midline shift to the right
5. Midline shift to the left
6. Left frontal lobe mass with bleeding
7. Right frontal lobe mass with infarction
8. Subarachnoid haemorrhage

(b) **What could be the diagnosis?**

1. Cerebral astrocytoma
2. Medulloblastoma
3. Intracranial bleed secondary to AV malformation
4. Cerebral abscess
5. Cerebral infarction
6. Benign increased intracranial pressure

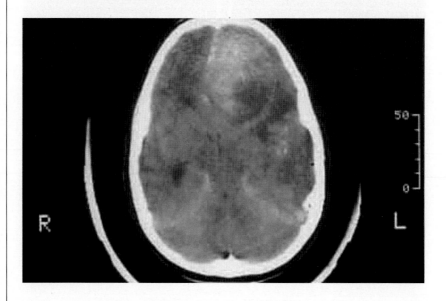

Case 119

This newborn infant was noted to have an abnormally shaped head with absent sutures. Her hands showed partially fused second and third fingers.

(a) **What are the abnormalities seen on examination of the head and face?**

    1. Epicanthic folds
    2. Midfacial hypoplasia
    3. Low frontal hairline
    4. Frontal prominence
    5. Prominent ear crus
    6. Micrognathia

(b) **What is a possible diagnosis?**

    1. Down's syndrome
    2. Apert's syndrome
    3. Saethre–Chotzen craniosynostosis
    4. Patau's syndrome
    5. Normal

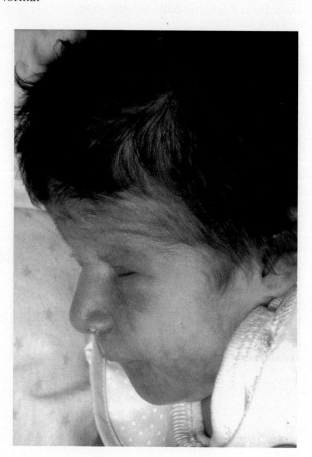

Case 120

A newborn term infant was noted to be cyanosed on examination, but there were no other abnormalities on cardiac or respiratory examination. Arterial blood gas was normal apart from a low pO_2. A hyperoxia test failed to improve the infant's saturation above 85%. The infant had a chest X-ray and echocardiogram.

(a) **What abnormalities are seen from these investigations?**

1. Dextrocardia
2. Rotated film
3. Cardiac failure
4. Pulmonary oligaemia
5. Parallel great vessels

(b) **Following diagnosis, what would be your immediate management?**

1. Prescribe furosemide
2. Start prostaglandin E_1 infusion
3. Intravenous antibiotics
4. Arrange for a Blalock–Taussig shunt
5. Arrange for a Rashkind balloon septostomy

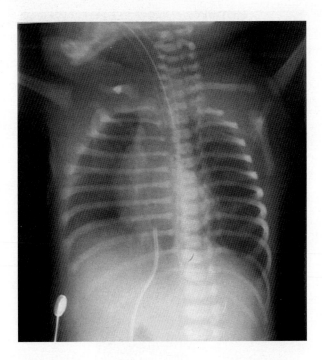

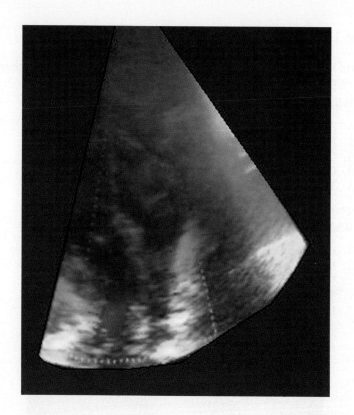

Case 121

A term infant had a choking episode on his feed. Each time a further feed was offered he would become dusky. A chest X-ray is perfomed.

(a) **What diagnoses is the chest X-ray consistent with?**

1. Aspiration
2. Right pulmonary hypoplasia
3. Cardiac failure
4. Oesophageal atresia
5. Tracheo-oesophageal fistula

Following the chest X-ray, he undergoes further investigations.

(b) **What is the investigation pictured and what does it show?**

1. Oesophagram demonstrating a tracheo-oesophageal fistula
2. Barium swallow demonstrating gastro-oesophageal reflux
3. CT scan of neck showing laryngeal web
4. Tomogram demonstrating vascular ring
5. Barium swallow demonstrating oesophageal atresia

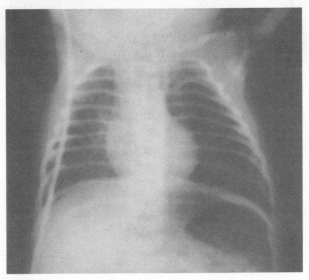

(a)

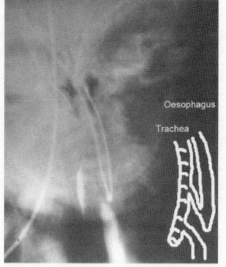

Oesophagus

Trachea

(b)

Case 122

This is a 6-month-old baby boy with a history of failure to thrive and vomiting. His blood test shows iron-deficiency anaemia; Igs TFT, chromosomes, lactate, ammonia, amino acids, organic acids, sweat test, coeliac screen, serum glucose and blood gas are all within normal ranges. The isotransferrin level is abnormally low.

(a) **What three abnormalities are seen on these two photographs?**

    1. Short upper limbs
    2. Multiple small haemangiomas
    3. Lipoatrophy
    4. Abnormal fat distribution on buttocks
    5. Flexed fixed deformities of limbs
    6. Inverted nipple

(b) **What is the diagnosis?**

    1. Refsum disease
    2. Zellweger's syndrome
    3. Hunter's syndrome
    4. Hypothyroidism
    5. Carbohydrate-deficient glycoprotein syndrome
    6. Glycogen storage disease type Ia

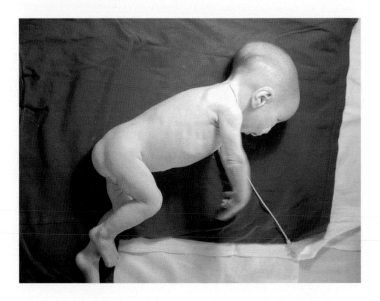

Case 123

A 12-year-old boy attends A&E with a 2-week history of pain in the neck and numbness over the volar aspect of his right forearm. Examination reveals tenderness over the upper thoracic midline region of his spine and difficulty gripping with his right hand. He undergoes a chest X-ray and thoracic MRI.

(a) **What abnormalities are seen?**

    1. Right hilar lymphadenopathy
    2. Right upper lobe pneumonia
    3. Paravertabral mass
    4. Mediastinal mass
    5. None

(b) **What further investigations would you perform?**

    1. Myelogram
    2. Heaf test
    3. Bronchoscopy
    4. Biopsy
    5. Sputum analysis

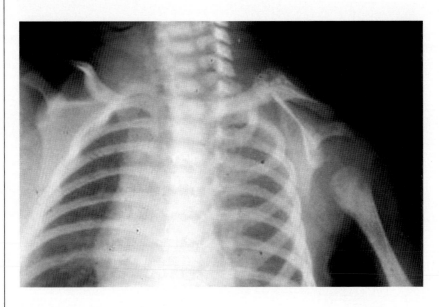

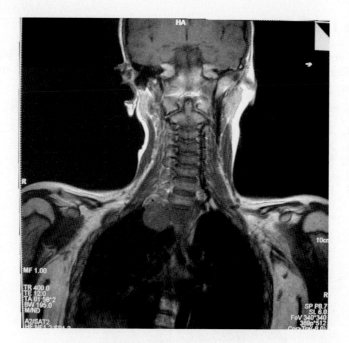

Case 124

A 15-year-old boy was referred by his GP with a history of night sweats, swelling in the neck and increasing difficulty in breathing over a 2-month period.

(a) **What investigations would you perform to obtain a diagnosis?**

1. Thyroid function tests
2. Mantoux test
3. Monospot
4. CT scan
5. Biopsy

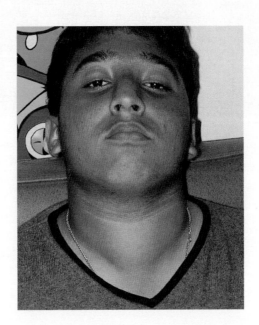

The boy undergoes lung function testing with a spirometer. The following printout is obtained, including a flow–volume loop:

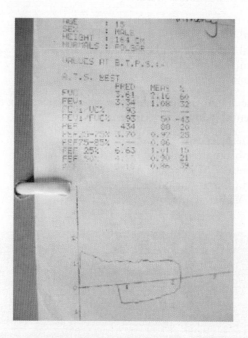

(b) **With which of these diagnoses are the results consistent?**

1. Asthma
2. Thyroid goitre
3. Cystic fibrosis
4. Mediastinal lymphoma
5. Scoliosis

Case 125

(a) **What is the abnormality here?**

1. Periventricular calcification
2. Bilateral dilated lateral ventricles
3. Bilateral subependymal calcification
4. Intraventricular calcification
5. Left frontal lobe mass

(b) **What is the diagnosis if the child has seizures, learning difficulties and developmental delay with skin lesions?**

1. Tuberous sclerosis
2. Neurofibromatosis type 1
3. Congenital CMV infection
4. Congenital toxoplasmosis
5. Sturge–Weber syndrome

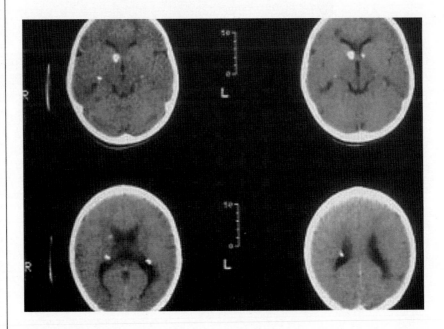

Case 101

Answers: (a) 1, 4, 5, 6
(b) 1, 4, 5

Cystic lesion following pneumonia

The main organisms causing cystic lesions following pneumonia are *S. aureus*, *Klebsiella* spp., *P. aeruginosa* and *Mycobacterium* spp. It is important to know the causative organism as well as to follow up with another X-ray in 6 weeks' time. Congenital adenomatous malformation of the lung is another diagnosis that should be considered if frequent infections occur on the same side. Bronchiectasis is rarely seen these days, but suspicion should be raised if frequent chest infection occurs. Chest CT can be very helpful in these cases, as can bronchoscopy (especially if a foreign body is suspected).

Case 102

Answers: (a) 2, 4, 6, 8
(b) 1, 2, 3, 5

Failure to thrive

Children who are not gaining weight and are having a problem achieving their milestones should be investigated. Detailed history-taking and full examination are very important before performing any tests. Infection is the first possibility that needs to be ruled out (such as urinary), and it is important to determine the calorie intake with the help of a dietician. If the child is not on solids and only on milk then baseline studies should be performed to evaluate thyroid function and determine the level of reducing substances in the urine. If the child is on solids then a coeliac screen should be added, together with a full blood count and measurement of blood haematinics. Calcium and bone biochemistry, together with liver function testing, should also be undertaken. A sweat test should be considered. After the first line of testing has been completed and the child is still not gaining weight, it is necessary to check immune function, check for allergies, and carry out a basic metabolic screen. Acid–base status should be checked to exclude a renal tabular problem. A cranial ultrasound scan if the fontanels are open will screen for a cerebral tumour. Early follow-up is essential. If initial tests are negative then the child should be admitted and feeding observed on the ward. A trial of nasogastric feeding may be necessary. Most cases of failure to thrive do not have any obvious cause. It is important to have a low threshold for considering abuse or neglect.

Case 103

Answers: (a) 3

(b) 3

Anal fissure

This is common in children with constipation either when it does not respond to treatment or when there is poor compliance with treatment. It can happen at any place around the anus. Children experiencing pain will not open their bowels even if the stools are soft. By the time the fissure heals, stools are becoming harder, and stimulants and softeners will cause large amounts of stool to pass through the anus – which will cause the fissure to reappear. It is important to treat pain with local analgesia, at the same time giving anticonstipation medication. In children with sexual abuse, there may be signs of additional perianal trauma and anal gaping is very prominent. Inflammatory bowel diseases may cause fissure – but very rarely.

Case 104

Answers: (a) 4

(b) 1, 2, 3

Orbital cellulitis

The spread of infection is usually from a paranasal sinus. The origin is most often from ethmoid sinuses in infants or ethmoid, frontal and maxillary sinuses in older children. It usually develops rapidly and can cause a high temperature, lethargy and leucocytosis, and the child may feel unwell and appear septic. If not treated rapidly and aggressively then complications may occur, including meningitis, cavernous sinus thrombosis and papilloedema. Preseptal cellulitis is usually associated with swollen eyelids and erythema around the eye. Septal involvement is associated with congested sclera, painful eye movements and swollen eyelids. In septal orbital cellulitis cranial CT should be considered when looking for a cause, as well as periorbital collections.

Case 105

Answers: (a) 2, 4

(b) 2, 5

Bilateral vesico-ureteric reflux with partial right duplex system

This can be complete with separate pelvis, separate ureter, and separate ureteric orifices. Or it can be incomplete with two pelvises and one ureter or two ureter united in a 'Y' shape. There is an increased risk of vesico-ureteric reflux, which leads to recurrent infection. Duplex kidneys are among the most common abnormalities detected on renal imaging, and in the absence of any problem no further action should be taken. If there is reflux then it is often from the ureter draining the lower moiety of the kidney and leading to the upper ureteric orifices. Partial nephrectomy can sometimes be performed if this part is badly scarred. If there is ureterocoele then this may cause obstruction and hydronephrosis as well.

Case 106

Answers: (a) 1
       (b) 1, 4

Intracranial injury (shaken baby syndrome)

This may be due to direct trauma or violent shaking. Direct trauma may be accidental, but children do not often injure themselves until they become independently mobile. Rolling off a bed or climbing out of a cot do not commonly cause skull fractures. A simple parietal fracture requires a fall of at least 1 metre to occur. Skull fractures that are complicated and multiple arouse the suspicion of non-accidental injury. Growing fractures with subdural haematoma and oedema are all more common in non-accidentally injured children than in others. About half of children with subdural haematomas will have no skull fracture or any bruises. Retinal haemorrhage is associated with shaken baby syndrome, and ophthalmological examination is required in suspected cases of non-accidental injury. Shaking causes shearing of vessels across the subdural space, and in cases of non-accidental injury subdural haemorrhage is seen characteristically in the posterior interhemispheric fissure. Neurological, intellectual and visual impairment occur in these babies.

Case 107

Answers: (a) 4, 5, 7
       (b) 3, 7, 8
       (c) 3

Craniopharyngioma

This is associated with growth retardation as a presenting feature as well as visual disturbances in children and failure of sexual maturation in adolescents. Bitemporal hemianopia is present in half of patients and homonymous hemianopia in 20%. Visual acuity is diminished in one or both eyes. Half of these children will have hydrocephalus causing headache and papilloedema. Hypothalamic involvement will cause diabetes insipidus and other endocrine dysfunction. If the tumour extends anteriorly, it may compress the olfactory tract causing anosmia, while lateral extension can cause 3rd and 4th cranial nerve palsy. Cranial MRI is important to localize the tumour for surgery and subtotal resection followed by radiotherapy. Hormone replacement therapy is needed. The prognosis is not usually very good, even with surgery, as total resection is not possible.

Case 108

Answer: 2

Management of tension pneumothorax

Tension pneumothorax is an emergency condition and if clinically suspected an urgent X-ray should be taken. If the patient's condition does not allow this then a chest drain should be inserted very quickly. There is no place for a butterfly needle in the management of tension pneumothorax except when chest drainage is not possible, because of the risk of creating a hole in the lung and thus causing a bronchopleural fistula. Analgesia and sedation should be given while the drain is still in place. The 2nd intercostal space outside the midclavicular line and the 4th intercostal space on the midaxillary line are the sites commonly used for drainage in neonates and both can be used in older children. The chest drain is connected to an underwater seal, and as long as bubbling continues, the drain should be kept in place. When bubbling stops, the drain should be clamped for 24 hours and chest X-ray repeated to confirm the absence of recurrence.

Case 109

Answers: (i) 1, 2, 3

(ii) 3

Coeliac disease

This is caused by exposure of the small intestine to the gluten component found in wheat, rye, barley and oats, leading to malabsorption. Presentation can be at any age, but usually between ages 9 and 18 months with failure to thrive, loose stools, anorexia and poor weight gain. Insidious iron-deficiency anaemia in older children can also be part of the presentation. If it is not picked up early, the infant will look thin, with a large belly and loss of muscle bulk in the legs and buttocks. The blood test may show iron-deficiency anaemia, anti-gliadin IgA antibodies will be positive and anti-endomysial and anti-reticulin antibodies will also be raised. The diagnosis should be confirmed with jejunal biopsy, and this must be done before diet exclusion (which will be for life). If there is no improvement on a gluten-free diet then the diagnosis of coeliac disease should be revised.

Case 110

Answers: (a) 1, 3, 4

　　　　(b) 1, 2, 4, 5

Juvenile chronic arthritis

The onset is usually at ages under 16 years. The symptoms should continue for a minimum of 3 months. There are three forms: systemic onset, polyarticular and pauciarticular. The systemic onset form occurs under the age of 5 years, with a toxic-looking child, who is irritable, with fever, splenomegaly, lymphadenopathy and arthritis affecting small joints. The temperature is intermittent up to 40°C. A large number of children have a maculopapular coppery red rash. There is no definitive laboratory test, but the white cell count will be high, as will platelets. The erythrocyte sedimentation rate is usually high. Rheumatoid factor is absent and antinuclear antibodies may be raised. The polyarticular form usually involves more than four joints – mainly large joints, and the neck, interphalangeal and metatarsal joints can be involved. It is usually bilateral and symmetrical. Ten percent of patients will have positive rheumatoid factor; this mainly affects girls and can be damaging.

Case 111

Answers: (a) 2, 3, 4, 5

　　　　(b) 3

Moya moya disease

This is a slowly progressive bilateral occlusion of the internal carotid arteries. The basilar artery is sometimes occluded as well. Multiple anastomoses have time to form between internal and external carotid arteries. The result is a new vascular network at the base of the brain. Symptoms can initially range from recurrent headache to abrupt hemiparesis. Sudden hemiplegia can affect the face and limbs. Aphasia, hemianopia and lethargy can be observed. Recovery will occur, but new attacks will start, and most patients are left with chronic weakness on one side, epilepsy and mental retardation. Transient ischaemic attacks are another presentation. Large infarcts can be seen on cranial CT. Definitive diagnosis can be by MRA or arteriography. Verapamil has been reported to be of some benefit. Surgical intervention is another way of management, but nothing is completely successful.

Case 112

Answers: (a) 1, 5

(b) 3

Aicardi's syndrome

This X-linked dominant condition occurs exclusively in girls and is associated with infantile spasms. It is characterized by infantile spasms and global developmental delay. Coloboma of the optic nerve, microphthalmia, microcephaly and vertebrocostal abnormalities occur in 50% of patients. The outcome is poor, with seizures and mental retardation. The corpus callosum is absent in all cases, and periventricular heterotopias and a dysplastic cortex are features on the MRI scan. Choroidoretinal lacunae are a prominent feature of this syndrome.

Case 113

Answers: (a) 4

(b) 1, 5

Skull fractures

More than 30% of children admitted with head injury will have a skull fracture. Few will develop an intracranial bleed. Most skull fractures are linear and the risk of extradural haematoma is low. Neonates' skulls are poorly mineralized membranous bone and fracture easily. Linear fractures due to birth trauma are rare. Skull fractures do not heal by callus and it is difficult to date them. They normally heal in 2–3 months. Sometimes there is no bruising at all over the scalp, even with a severe impact. It is important to recognize depressed skull fractures and refer to a neurosurgeon. Compound fractures due to penetrating injury can be very serious. Very rarely children will develop basal skull fractures. There is controversy regarding the need for skull X-rays in the event of head trauma. When child abuse is suspected or in the case of depressed fractures, there may be an indication. Where conciousness has been impaired or any fluid is coming from the ears or nose, cranial CT should be performed.

Case 114

Answers: (a) (i) 1
          (ii) 5
         (iii) 3
     (b) (i) 1
          (ii) 2
         (iii) 2, 8

Otitis media

This occurs in infants and children as the eustachian tube is shorter, wider and more horizontal than in adults. The presence of adenoids in children and their proximity to the eustachian tube makes children more vulnerable to acute otitis media. It is always accompanied by upper respiratory tract infection. Painful ears with bilaterality is the most common presentation. The child will develop fever, and otitis media is one of the causes of febrile convulsions. The eardrum will appear red and acutely inflamed. Sometimes the tympanic membrane is bulging due to fluid collection. This will cause more pain and the infant will cry inconsolably. If the membrane ruptures then either clear fluid or pus will discharge and usually dry within 2–3 days. The drum will heal, and analgesia, antipyretics and antibiotics will help. In infants and children with recurrent otitis media, grommet insertion will help to prevent chronic otitis media and deafness. In older children, removal of the adenoids will help to reduce the recurrence of otitis media.

Case 115

Answer: 5

Human bites

Bites cause two hemispherical bruises with superimposed marks outlining the position of teeth. They can be matched against dental impressions of suspected assailants. Specialist help from a forensic dental surgeon should be sought. Photographs should be taken at presentation and social service involvement should be sought early on.

Case 116

Answers: (a) 1, 4

(b) 3

Lissencephaly

This is a neuronal migration defect characterized by a complete absence of gyri, leading to a smooth brain surface. It is sporadic and most children present with developmental delay or intractable myoclonic seizures, including infantile spasms. Microcephaly is prominent and all children are mentally retarded. Axial hypotonia and poor development of milestones are prominent. The EEG will help in diagnosing the hypsarrhythmia with fast high-voltage dysrhythmic activity and abnormal background. MRI scan is abnormal, as is cranial CT. Ventricles are usually enlarged and sometimes the corpus callosum is absent. Seizures are intractable, but infantile spasms respond to vigabatrin and/or steroids in high dose. Death occurs early during infancy.

Case 117

Answers: (a) 2, 5, 7

(b) 2, 4, 5

Extradural collection

This is a localized collection of blood between the dura and skull and occurs in 1% of head trauma cases in children. The bleeding originates from the meningeal artery or its branches or from torn dural veins. Arterial bleeding results in a rapid progression of symptoms and signs. It is often associated with brain oedema, which increases the risk of a rise in intracranial pressure. With bleeding from veins, symptom progression is slower. More than 50% of bleeding occurs under the age of 2 years. It usually starts with loss of consciousness, followed by recovery and then rapid deterioration. In children this usually happens over hours, sometimes days. It takes the form of deterioration with loss of consciousness and the appearance of neurological signs (vomiting, papilloedema, 3rd nerve palsy, hemiparesis and retinal haemorrhage with a dilated fixed pupil on the side of collection being present in 90% of cases). Without treatment, the child will decerebrate and will go into a coma and die. Cranial CT is characterized by evidence of a convex area of increased density located immediately beneath the inner skull. Operative evacuation of the haematoma is the only way to save the child's life and should be done without delay. If the child is conscious and there is no neurological deficit then conservative treatment will be enough.

Case 118

Answers: (a) 1, 4, 6

(b) 1

Astrocytoma

This is divided into three grades: low-grade, anaplastic and glioblastoma multiforme. The presentation depends on the location of the tumour. It can be as seizures, hemiparesis or movement disorders. Seizures are the most common presenting features of low-grade gliomas. Tumours infiltrating the basal ganglia and internal capsule are less likely to present with seizures. Because of the slow growth of the tumour mass, signs and symptoms may not be obvious. Headache is common, occurring in the early morning in association with vomiting or nausea. More than 80% of patients at presentation with astrocytoma will have persisting headache, vomiting and nausea. Mass effect may cause cerebral oedema, midline shift and pressure on the aqueduct, resulting in non-communicating hydrocephalus. Neuroimaging is indicated in all children presenting with these symptoms. Dexamethasone should be given to reduce intracranial hypertension prior to surgery. Complete removal of the tumour is rarely possible except in cystic cerebral astrocytoma. The 5-year survival rate after surgery is 90% for low-grade and cystic astrocytomas. For anaplastic astrocytoma the 5-year survival rate is 30%, while for glioblastoma multiforme it is only 3%.

Case 119

Answers: (a) 2, 3, 4, 5

(b) 3

Saethre–Chotzen craniosynostosis

In this condition the predominant features are often evident at birth and include brachycephaly, midfacial hypoplasia, prominent ear crura and syndactyly. The coronal, lamboid and metopic sutures are fused. The condition is inherited in an autosomal dominant manner, with variable expression.

Premature craniosynostosis may be acquired after rickets or other metabolic conditions, or may be seen as part of an inherited/congenital syndrome. Generalized craniosynostosis, as in the above condition or in Crouzon's syndrome (where the coronal, sagittal and lamboidal sutures fuse), will cause a microcephalic deformity often associated with raised intracranial pressure, resulting in brain, optic and auditory nerve damage with consequences for normal neurodevelopment. Childern with these conditions need early referral to specialist cranio-facial units. Asymmetrical or localized premature fusion can cause different types of head shape, such as scaphocephaly (fusion of sagittal suture causing increased A-P growth) or brachycephaly (fusion of both coronal sutures causing flattening of the occiput). Plagiocephaly is caused by a unilateral synostosis of the coronal and occasionally lambdoid suture causing asymmetrical flattening of the parieto-occipital area. It has become more common with the 'back-to-sleep' advice. It rarely needs intervention as the deformity becomes less obvious as the child grows.

Case 120

Answers: (a) 1, 2, 5

(b) 2, 5

Transposition of the great vessels

The chest X-ray is rotated and does not provide a great deal of information on the aetiology of the infant's cyanosis. The lung fields and vascular markings are probably normal. An echocardiogram confirmed the diagnosis of transposition of the great arteries with a parallel side-by-side arrangement of the great vessels (pulmonary and aorta). The remainder of the scan was normal apart from the presence of a small patent ductus arteriosus. The immediate management was to maintain a shunt between the pulmonary and systemic circulations by starting a prostaglandin E_1 infusion to open the ductus arteriosus. The paediatric cardiologist performed a Rashkind balloon septostomy across the foramen ovale. The infant was then transferred to a paediatric cardiac surgical unit, where he underwent an arterial switch procedure.

Case 121

Answers: (a) 1, 5

(b) 1

Tracheo-oesophageal fistula

The initial chest X-ray is somewhat rotated but does show some increased shadowing in the right lung and upper lobes. A nasogastric tube was initially passed into the stomach, but the infant continued to have dusky episodes on oral feeding. An oesophagram demonstrated an oesophageal pouch and two tracheo-oesphageal fistulae in proximal and distal positions (see the sketch on image (b)). The infant was transferred to a paediatric surgical unit for correction. This type of fistula is very uncommon.

The commonest type of tracheo-oesophageal fistula is associated with a blind-ending proximal oesophagus and distal oesophageal tracheal fistula. There may be a normal air pattern in the bowel. During pregnancy there may be a history of hydramnios and soon after birth copious oral secretions may be observed. The diagnosis may be ascertained by observing the nasogastric tube to be coiled up in the oesophagus.

Case 122

Answers: (a) 4, 5, 6
        (b) 5

Carbohydrate-deficient glycoprotein syndrome

This comprises a group of inherited multisystem disorders characterized by a deficiency of carbohydrate moieties in a number of sialoproteins that are most readily detected in transferrin. There are four types, of which type I is the most frequent and is inherited in an autosomal recessive manner. All cases exhibit olivopontocerebellar atrophy and myelin-like lysosomal storage granules on electron microscopy. The infantile features of type I are poor feeding, failure to thrive, floppiness, gross motor delay with profound axial hypotonia, muscular weakness and later ataxia. Acquired microcephaly, weak tendon reflexes later becoming areflexia, visual intention, roving eye movements and internal strabismus are frequent. The majority of cases have facial dysmorphism, inverted nipples, joint restrictions, thoracic deformity, and unusual lipodystrophy with fat pads above the buttocks, perineal region and/or fingers. There are lipodystrophic streaks on the limbs and mild hepatomegaly. Fifty percent of patients develop epilepsy with low IQ and regression over the first 5 years of life. There is a marked reduction in tetrasialotransferrin and an increase in mono-, di- and trisialotransferrin.

Case 123

Answers: (a) 3
        (b) 2, 4

Primitive neuroectodermal tumour

The initial chest X-ray suggested right upper lobe pneumonia. However, MRI scanning demonstrated that the mass in the right upper zone of the lung was extrapleural and arising from the paravertebral region. The differential diagnosis was of a tuberculous mass (Pott's disease of the spine) or a malignancy. Following a negative Heaf test and the finding of normal inflammatory markers, this patient underwent an emergency decompression after developing signs of cord compression. Biopsy of the mass under general anaesthetic confirmed a diagnosis of primitive neuroectodermal tumour (PNET) involving infiltration of the T1 and T2 vertebrae. Resection was incomplete. PNETs are rapidly growing tumours frequently metastasizing via the CSF pathways to the spinal and cranial subarachnoid spaces and are highly malignant, both histologically and clinically. They are difficult to classify but most commonly arise in the cerebellum (medulloblastomas), but can arise in the pineal gland, cerebrum, spinal cord brain stem and peripheral nerves. Where total resection is incomplete, chemotherapy is used, sometimes with irradiation. The 5-year survival rate is only 40–60%.

Case 124

Answers: (a) 1, 2, 3, 4, 5
(b) 2, 4

Mediastinal lymphoma

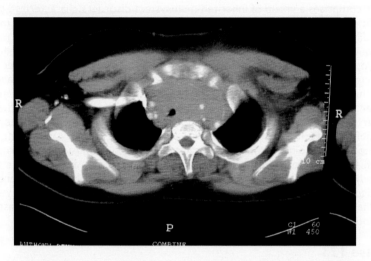

Although this boy had a pronounced swelling of his neck, a chest X-ray was not diagnostic. CT scan of his chest, however, showed an extensive mass extending from the neck into the mediastinum, compressing and deviating the trachea to the left. His thyroid function tests, Mantoux test, FBC and monospot were all normal. Biopsy of the mass in the neck confirmed a non-Hodgkin's lymphoma.

The pattern of his flow–volume loop obtained using a spirometer is consistent with large extra- and intrathoracic airway obstruction. On inspecting the expiratory loop, peak expiratory flow rate is markedly reduced, with an FEV1 30% PR. In contrast, the expiratory flow is relatively well preserved at lower lung volume, with FEF75 39% PR. Similarly, the early peak inspiratory flow rate is blunted. Expiratory flow rates in small-airway disease such as asthma or cystic fibrosis tend to have better predicted FEV1 compared with FEF75, with the pattern of the expiratory loop showing a scalloped appearance.

Case 125

Answers: (a) 3

         (b) 1

Tuberous sclerosis

This is transmitted as an autosomal dominant condition. It is the commonest neurocutaneous condition. Early presentation can be as seizures – mainly infantile spasms, but other types of seizure can be present. Developmental delay is a universal association with tuberous sclerosis. All children with mental retardation will have seizures. Hypopigmented, ash leaf and shagreen patches develop later. Other symptoms are hyperpigmented patches, periungual hamartomas, adenoma sebaceum on the face, phakomas in the retina, rhabdomyomas, renal hamartomas, kidney cysts, hamartomas of lungs and bone, subependymal tuberosity in the brain (which looks like periventricular calcification), and cortical tuberosity. Seizures are difficult to control; surgical excision of cortical tuberosities may reduce the seizure frequency if it has been shown that they are the source of the seizures.

Index of cases

WITHDRAWN FROM LIBRARY
LIBRARY · BRITISH MEDICAL ASSOCIATION